Law
Prac
Health Nursing

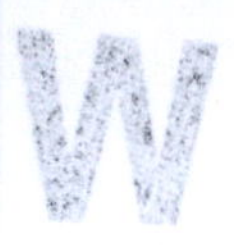

Law, Values and Practice in Mental Health Nursing

A handbook

Toby Williamson and Rowena Daw

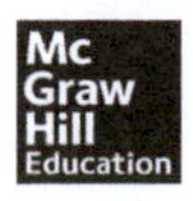

Open University Press

Open University Press
McGraw-Hill Education
McGraw-Hill House
Shoppenhangers Road
Maidenhead
Berkshire
England
SL6 2QL

email: enquiries@openup.co.uk
world wide web: www.openup.co.uk

and Two Penn Plaza, New York, NY 10121-2289, USA

First published 2013

A catalogue record of this book is available from the British Library

ISBN-13: 978-0-335-24501-7
ISBN-10: 0-335-24501-3
eISBN: 978-0-335-24502-4

Library of Congress Cataloging-in-Publication Data
CIP data applied for

Typeset by Aptara, Inc., India

Praise for this book

"I welcome this book as its integration of values based practice and legislation into the complex world of decision making in mental health services clarifies many issues. I found the hypothetical scenarios and reflection points along the way a very useful vehicle to achieve the careful consideration that such issues require. This book is sure to become essential reading for students of mental health nursing."
Ian Hulatt, Mental Health Advisor, Royal College of Nursing UK

"This is an invaluable guide for all professionals working in mental health services, written by two people who have unparalleled understanding of mental health and mental capacity law. It should help practitioners understand both the intricacies of the law and how to retain a person-centred approach when applying it."
Paul Farmer, Chief Executive, Mind

"An impressive and enlightening book that spans law, ethics, values and practice. With the help of realistic scenarios it explains and applies the law with clarity and great practical understanding. It will inform and reassure those struggling with the often painful dilemmas confronted over the course of providing nursing care to service users with mental disabilities."
Genevra Richardson, Professor of Law, King's College London, UK

Contents

Acknowledgements

The authors would like to thank Chris Heginbotham and Camilla Parker for helping develop the original structure of the book, Professor Bill Fulford for commenting on Chapter 5, Caroline Davis, Tom Hore and Simon Lawton-Smith for their assistance, and Paul Gantley OBE for expert advice.

Toby would like to thank Rowena for her hard work and enormous contribution to the book, the Mental Health Foundation for giving him time and support to write the book, and his wife Jane for her toleration and support of what has been a rather long-lasting saga and everyone else who gave him encouragement.

Rowena would like to thank Toby for his expert work and for his patience in coping with long-distance communication for the 6 months while she was abroad, and give thanks to Mrs Linnet Szmukler, Dr John Morgan and Dr Tony Zigmond for their professional advice and assistance with case scenarios.

Acronyms

AC	approved clinician
ADRT	advance decision to refuse treatment
AMHP	approved mental health professional
ANH	artificial nutrition and hydration
AWOL	absent without leave
BIA	best interests assessor
CAMHS	Child and Adolescent Mental Health Services
CBT	cognitive behavioural therapy
CPA	care programme approach
CPN	community psychiatric nurse
CQC	Care Quality Commission
CRPD	Convention on the Rights of Persons with Disabilities
CTO	community treatment order
DBT	dialectical behavioural therapy
DH	Department of Health
DoLS	Deprivation of Liberty Safeguards
EA	Equality Act
ECHR	European Convention on Human Rights
ECtHR	European Court of Human Rights
ECT	electro-convulsive therapy
EHRC	Equalities and Human Rights Commission
EPA	enduring power of attorney
EVB	evidence-based practice
HRA	Human Rights Act
IMCA	independent mental capacity advocate
IMHA	independent mental health advocate
LPA	lasting power of attorney
MCA	Mental Capacity Act
MDT	multidisciplinary team
MHA	Mental Health Act
NICE	National Institute for Health and Clinical Excellence
NMC	Nursing and Midwifery Council
NR	nearest relative
OPG	Office of the Public Guardian
PD	personality disorder
RC	responsible clinician
RCN	Royal College of Nursing
RPR	relevant person's representative

s	Section
SCIE	Social Care Institute for Excellence
SCT	supervised community treatment
SMT	serious medical treatment
SOAD	second opinion appointed doctor
UNCRC	UN Convention on the Rights of the Child
VBP	values-based practice

Introduction

There are no answers - only choices.

(From the film, *Solaris*)

Why this book is important: the law, policy and people

The law

This handbook is about mental health nursing and the law, focusing particularly on the Mental Capacity Act 2005 and the Mental Health Act 1983 (as amended in 2007).

The Mental Capacity Act (MCA) is an entirely new piece of legislation and came into force in 2007. Additional mental capacity legal safeguards, the Deprivation of Liberty Safeguards (DoLS) came into force in 2009. The amendments to the Mental Health Act (MHA), which are both extensive and important, came into force in 2008. They affect people with mental illnesses and other mental health problems (including personality disorders and other psychological disorders), 'organic' conditions such as dementia, alcohol or substance misuse problems, learning disabilities, learning difficulties, developmental disabilities (e.g. autism), or combinations of those illnesses, disabilities and conditions. For any mental health nurse working in England or Wales in hospital settings, residential care, or the community, there have not been such significant changes in the law since the original Mental Health Act came into force in 1983.

Policy

These changes in the law have also occurred at a time when mental health problems, and conditions such as dementia, have been the focus of much greater attention from policy-makers and service providers. This has partly been an acknowledgement of the relative neglect of mental health in general, of people with mental illnesses and of mental health services, as compared with physical health, and physical health services that treat them.

In 1999, the Department of Health published the National Service Framework (NSF) for Mental Health for England (Department of Health 1999) which led to a substantial increase in funding for mental health services over the next ten years. This built upon the shift from hospital-based care to community care and the development of new types of community services to provide that care. In 2004, the government's Social Exclusion Unit's publication, *Mental Health and Social Exclusion and Mental Health* (Social Exclusion Unit 2004) focused on the social impact of mental ill health, including the significant social exclusion and discrimination such people may face. A new mental health strategy to replace the NSF was published in 2011, *No Health Without Mental Health* (Department of Health 2011).

In 2009, the Department of Health published *Living Well with Dementia*, England's first national dementia strategy that resulted in increased investment in dementia services (Department of Health 2009a). Wales has given a similar priority to mental health and dementia and at the time of writing was consulting on its new mental health strategy that includes dementia. Services for people with learning disabilities have also had greater attention paid to them with the publication of *Valuing People* by the Department of Health in 2001, and its follow-up strategy *Valuing People Now* in 2009 (Department of Health 2009b).

Recently, other policies have perhaps had a bigger bearing on mental health services, most notably the restrictions and reductions in public spending. This has put added pressure on staff working in these services but the economic situation that has given rise to them is unlikely to reduce the demand on those services. It may even increase the pressure as unemployment, homelessness, growing inequalities, and social deprivation impact upon individuals' mental health. We are also living in an ageing society with more people growing older and living longer than ever before. While depression and dementia are not inevitable consequences of growing old (dementia, as well as depression, affects people under the age of 65), for those in later life the risk of becoming depressed or getting some form of dementia certainly does increase with age.

People

At any point in time one in six people in the UK is experiencing some form of mental distress and one in four people will experience it at some point in their lives. Some 25 per cent of people over the age of 65 have symptoms of depression severe enough to warrant therapeutic intervention and one in five people over the age of 80 have some form of dementia. At least 1 million people in England and Wales may lack the capacity to make certain decisions because of a mental illness, dementia or learning disability and over 4 million people are involved in their support and care, either as families and friends, or in a paid role. These are very substantial numbers of people and although many will never have contact with mental health nurses or be directly affected by the law, a significant number will. Unless otherwise stated, by around 2010 in England and Wales the following numbers were valid:

- 10,627,500 people have a functional mental disorder (nearly 1 in 5 of the population).
- 685,900 people have some form of dementia. Two-thirds live in the community.
- 9,456,300 adults drink over the recommended safe limits for alcohol.
- 3,000,000 adults used illicit drugs.
- 918,800 people have a learning disability.
- 192,968 people with mental illness, dementia, learning disabilities, alcohol or substance misuse were admitted to psychiatric hospital.

- 44,535 people were detained in hospital under the Mental Health Act in 2010–11. 16,647 people were being detained in England on 31 March 2011.
- 312,478 people with mental illness, dementia, learning disabilities, alcohol or substance misuse live in residential care homes.
- 3,258 people were subject to supervised community treatment in 2010–11 under the Mental Health Act 1983.
- 5,228 people who lacked mental capacity were subject to a Deprivation of Liberty Safeguards authorisation under the Mental Capacity Act 2005 in 2010–11.
- There were 10,680 situations involving an Independent Mental Capacity Advocate (IMHA) in 2010–11 in England.
- People detained under the Mental Health Act 1983 had regular access to an IMHA on 65 per cent of 311 psychiatric wards surveyed in 2009–10.

For those people who do have contact with mental health nurses and the MCA or MHA, the experience will be unique to the individual and they must be treated with the respect, sensitivity and care that one would expect to receive in a similar situation. The experience may involve considerable distress because of the illness, condition or disability giving cause for a legal intervention, and also the person not understanding or consenting to the care or treatment being provided through that intervention.

Legislation can be daunting. Mental health nurses want their practice to be legal and ethical. Nurses do not want to break the law or get it wrong. At times, however, they may be required by the law, or need to use the law, to provide care and treatment to someone who is unable or unwilling to give their consent. This can feel stressful, uncomfortable or even upsetting but will be a requirement of the job at times, and refusing to be involved in these situations is not acceptable. Mental health nurses can, therefore, understandably feel worried about the legislation and major changes in legislation that affect their practice. It is crucial that they understand them. This book enables nurses to reach that understanding.

Why this book is important: nursing practice and the law

People with mental health problems or other conditions which may affect their ability to make decisions about their care and treatment may, like nurses, also be very worried, upset or frightened when the law is used to allow things to be done to them that they don't understand or believe are necessary. It is not at all uncommon to hear someone say, that 'they haven't done anything wrong' or 'they haven't broken the law' as a protest when the MHA is being used to restrain or detain them (especially if the police are involved). Family members and friends may share this view. And even where someone is unaware of the law being used, such as gently restraining a person with dementia who is about to put themselves in danger, they may respond with physical aggression. The wrong response by a nurse may lead to a contravention of the person's legal rights. That is why it is also essential that nurses understand how to apply the legislation correctly in practice.

Difficult issues of compulsion, control, and the rights of patients arise much more frequently in mental health nursing. Nurses need to be equipped with the right set of skills to deal with the ethical tensions that arise in providing good quality care and treatment which remain both lawful and respectful of the different perspectives and values that patients may hold. This is particularly important where nurses are working in areas containing diverse ethnic, religious and cultural communities.

A number of books on mental health law have been written for legal professionals or for practitioners with specific roles defined by the law (e.g. approved mental health professionals). Some textbooks give detailed legal descriptions of the two laws but are not expansive in explaining how they apply in practice. Nor do they explain fully the crucial interface between the laws and situations where they may both apply at the same time. There is currently no book aimed exclusively at mental health nurses explaining how the MCA and the MHA apply to their everyday practice, including situations where both laws apply at the same time. This handbook aims to do exactly that. It also explains the relevance of the Human Rights Act and the Equality Act, both of which have a direct bearing on practice, and it includes policies and protocols such as the Care Programme Approach.

Why this book is important: values, nursing practice, and the law

This handbook also explains how the two laws should work within a framework of 'values-based practice'. Values-based practice is not a requirement of either law, nor is it referred to in either of them. But to be a good mental health nurse it is essential to understand the relationship between values and ethics and the correct application of the law, particularly where an individual does not understand, agree or decide about being detained and/or treated without their consent. Situations like this may generate differences of opinion and conflict involving a nurse, a service user, a family carer, and other practitioners, require clear and calm communication, and an ability and understanding of what the legislation means in practice. It may be difficult to decide the best course of action, what are the most important principles to uphold (typically, service user's autonomy or freedom versus protection and public safety), or even which law should be used. Simply following the letter of the law, like an instruction manual, is likely to prove insufficient in dealing with these complex issues. Values-based practice provides a very useful process for working through these complexities and keeping people, rather than legal procedures, at the centre of what one does.

So this handbook is about people – nurses, people with mental illnesses, problems, conditions, dependencies, people with learning disabilities, their families and friends, other professionals and staff, advocates, and wider communities.

The authors have extensive practical and theoretical experience of mental heath legislation, including frontline experience of managing mental health services. The challenge of working legally and ethically with people potentially subject to mental health or mental capacity legislation can appear daunting but in our experience it is perhaps the most fulfilling and rewarding area of practice. This is because, when done well, it necessitates using all one's skills, expertise and experience in working with individuals: involvement, negotiation, respect for the individual, good communication, multi-disciplinary (and multi-agency) working, a tolerance of uncertainty, working with difference and diversity, ability to manage power imbalances fairly, honesty, and compassion. When done well, it not only protects people's rights but in most cases may also assist in a person's recovery, improve their quality of life, or provide them with opportunities to regain control over their illness, or disability.

A word about the law

The law is important to all nurses who practise in mental health. First comes the Human Rights Act, a kind of superior law that all other laws (legislation and common law) must comply with. It provides a framework of individual rights and freedoms, which nurses working in all fields of mental health must follow. The Mental Health Act 1983 (MHA) and the Mental Capacity Act 2005 (MCA), together with their Codes of Practice, govern the care and treatment of all services users, in the case of the MCA and particular patients in the case of the MHA. The common law also applies to some matters, like consent to treatment.

In this book we refer regularly to sections of the MCA or the MHA, to the Codes of Practice and occasionally to the common law and to court cases. So, a word about the law generally. The MHA and the MCA started life as Bills before Parliament. Civil servants drew them up after consultations with the public and groups of people who were directly involved. This included the NHS and local authorities but also an immensely wide range of people who have a stake in the laws: service users and their families, carers, nurses, psychiatrists, social workers, occupational therapists, care home managers, people working in the criminal justice system like the police and courts, and the voluntary organisations who represent people with mental health problems, learning disabilities, dementia and aged care. All Bills are debated and pass through both Houses of Parliament before they become statutes. Sometimes, as with the recent 2007 Mental Health Act, they do not come into force immediately or different parts come into force at different times.

Because Scotland, Northern Ireland and Wales have the power to make their own laws on some matters, not all the laws passed by the Westminster Parliament apply to them. While the Human Rights Act applies throughout the UK, the MHA and the MCA only apply to England and Wales. Recently Wales has been granted wide law-making powers in mental health and the Welsh Assembly has already made some changes to the MHA which now apply only in Wales.

Statutes

Statutes like the MCA and the MHA are divided into different Parts, consisting of sections setting out the rules. They contain schedules at the end that set out more detail about how the law will operate. The statutes provide the general powers, duties, rights and safeguards of the law. *Powers* are what specified individuals (for instance, doctors and nurses) *may* lawfully do under the statute, *duties* are what they *must* do, and *rights* are what specified people (like patients and carers) are entitled to and can (usually) make a legal case about if they do not get them. A 'safeguard' is a term for the rights and systems of rules that are there to protect persons subject to the law. In the case of mental health and mental capacity, it is important that the statute has a balance between the powers and duties of the professionals and the safeguards for the patients and their carers. This will become clearer in a later chapter when we spell out how the MHA and the MCA work.

Regulations

Regulations are drawn up by civil servants and are laid before Parliament but are then passed without detailed debate. They are more flexible than statutes because they can be changed by the same simple process. Statutes, however, can only be changed by the full parliamentary process.

Codes of Practice

Codes of Practice are produced in the same way as Regulations except that they always involve extensive consultation before being laid before Parliament. Unlike statutes or regulations, they are not strictly binding but they are more than mere guidance or good practice. Professionals and others operating the Codes must 'have regard' to the Codes, and courts and tribunals must take account of them in deciding individual cases. They should always be followed unless there is a very good reason not to do so in the particular case, or because of a policy for a class of cases. Failure to follow the Code of Practice can be illegal if the court does not believe there was a 'cogent reason' to depart from the Code (see R (Munjaz) v Mersey Care NHS Trust [2006] AC 148).

Both the MCA and the MHA are accompanied by sets of Regulations and Codes of Practice, including a Code of Practice for DoLS. The Welsh Ministers have published a separate Code of Practice for the MHA in Wales.

The common law

The common law is the term for the rules laid down by judges in individual cases in areas of law that are not governed by statute. There is a hierarchy in the courts. If a case comes before one of the higher courts (High Court, Court of Appeal or the Supreme Court) and they make a decision of principle, that principle becomes an established part of the law unless another court higher up the system changes it. Judges also make binding decisions about the meaning of statutes and in that way they can change how a statute is interpreted in the future.

How to use this book

This book is divided into two parts. Part I provides an overview of the MCA and the MHA, as well as brief summaries of the Human Rights Act and Equality Act. It also contains a chapter describing values-based practice. If you just need a quick reference guide to these laws, or want to understand more about values-based practice, you can do this by going to the relevant chapter in Part I. The chapters contain scenarios, many based upon real-life situations that the authors have been involved with, to illustrate key issues, as well as references to relevant research and other guidance, reflection points and exercises that readers can do to gain a better understanding of applying the law in practice.

Part II goes into more detail about how the two laws apply in practice, referring to values-based practice wherever appropriate. It has been written to try and take into account all the main settings that mental health nurses may work in, and the most common situations that may arise where the MCA and/or the MHA may apply. The chapters therefore follow a number of 'journeys' or 'encounters' involving different people as they come into contact with services provided by mental health nurses, and identifying the relevant pieces of legislation at each stage. The journeys and encounters involve people with different mental health problems, illnesses, conditions and disabilities in order to comprehensively illustrate the different aspects of the legislation. The chapters in Part II begin with people living in the community who are coming into contact with mental health services for the first time, follow people through hospital admission, care, treatment and discharge, and then look at people in residential care, and children and young people.

At the end of this book is a list of Useful Resources and an Appendix containing a decision matrix as a quick reference guide to the conditions of use of the MCA and the MHA.

A note on coverage of more general and specific issues

This book is an introductory text to mental health law, policy and related practice but it is not comprehensive. We do not have space to deal with all the important but general issues for mental health nurses, in particular regarding confidentiality and information sharing, risk assessment and prescribing practice for psychiatric drugs. It is understood that these core issues will be taught as a general part of nursing training.

We are also unable to consider in depth specialised areas which may have a bearing on the path a detained person takes through the health system, for example, forensic patients' relationships with the criminal justice system and the transition of young people to adult services. Knowledge of these broader issues should be gained once a nurse decides to specialise in these areas.

A note on geographical coverage

The MCA and the MHA only apply in England and Wales. Scotland has its own mental health and mental capacity legislation: the Mental Health (Care and Treatment) (Scotland) Act 2003 and the Adults with Incapacity (Scotland) Act 2000. Northern Ireland has its own separate Mental Health Order (made in 1986, and largely replicating the provisions of the MHA 1983) but no mental capacity legislation at the time of writing (though it plans to introduce a new unified mental health and mental capacity law in the future). This book therefore only applies to mental health nurses practising in England and Wales.

A note on language

This book is about people who have contact with mental health nurses, and how the law affects them. However, the law, codes of practice, policy, guidance, and personal and ideological preferences have resulted in a range of terms existing to refer to people, including 'patients', 'service users', 'clients', even 'P' (meaning 'person lacking capacity') or 'he' (not 'she') in the MCA. Similarly, there are a range of terms to describe what may cause someone to have contact with mental health nurses including 'mental health problems', 'mental illnesses', 'disorders' or 'impairments', 'conditions', 'disabilities' and 'diseases' (e.g. Alzheimer's disease). Our preference as authors would always be to refer to the person first, and then the reason for their contact with a nurse (e.g. 'person with mental health problems', 'person with dementia') but unfortunately this is often too cumbersome or does not easily fit with the particular context or situation. At different times in this book different terms may therefore be used depending on the context, to ensure simplicity of explanation, or to provide consistency with what the law or official guidance says. We hope the reader understands why and it is not interpreted as us labelling or demeaning the individuals or issues involved.

In everyday practice we would urge all mental health nurses to try and use language that the people they are treating or caring for understand, and at best can positively relate to or at worst, do not actively reject as being irrelevant or offensive. As advocates for the people you work with, we would also encourage you to try and persuade your colleagues to do the same.

Sources for statistics

Alzheimer's Society (2011) *Mapping the Dementia Gap*. London: Alzheimer's Society.

Care Quality Commission, *Monitoring the Mental Health Act in 2010/11.*

Department of Health, *Hospital Episode Statistics Online, 2010–11, England.*

Department of Health (2011) *Report for Health and Social Care, 2010–11.*

Health Inspectorate Wales, *Deprivation of Liberty Safeguards Annual Monitoring.*

Home Office, *Drugs Strategy, 2010.*

Improving Health and Lives Learning Disabilities Observatory, *People with Learning Disabilities in England, 2011: Services and Support.*

London School of Economics (2007) *Dementia UK.*

NHS Information Centre (2009) *Adult Psychiatric Morbidity in England, 2007: Results of a Household Survey.*

NHS Information Centre (2011a) *Mental Capacity Act 2005, Deprivation of Liberty Safeguards Assessments (England): Second Report on Annual Data, 2010–11.*

NHS Information Centre (2011b) *Community Care Statistics: Social Services Activity. England, 2010–11: Provisional Release.*

NHS Information Centre (2011c) *NHS Mental Health Minimum Dataset, 2010–11, Admission of Patients to Mental Health Facilities, 2010–11: In-patients Formally Detained in Hospitals under the Mental Health Act 1983, Annual Figures, England, 2010/11.*

Office of National Statistics, *General Lifestyle Survey, 2009*.
Public Health Wales Observatory, *Profiles of Lifestyle and Health, 2010*.
Statistics for Wales, *National Dementia Action Plan for Wales, 2011; Local Authority Registers of People with Disabilities at 31 March 2010*.
The Fourth Year of the Independent Mental Capacity Advocacy (IMCA) Service, 2010–2011.
Welsh Government, *Substance Misuse in Wales, 2010–11*.
Welsh Government, *Welsh Health Survey, 2011: Initial Headline Results*.
Welsh Government Statistics, *Admission of Patients to Mental Health Facilities, 2010–11*.

Part I
The law, values and ethics

Introduction

Part I provides an overview of the MCA and MHA, as well as brief summaries of the Human Rights Act and Equality Act. It also contains a chapter describing values-based practice. If you need just a quick reference guide to the MCA or MHA, or want to understand a bit more about values-based practice, you can do this by going to the relevant chapter in this part of the book.

Understanding how the MCA, MHA and DoLS fit together

One of the most difficult aspects of understanding how legislation applies to day-to-day nursing practice is knowing which law applies in which situation, how the MCA (including DoLS) and MHA 'fit' with each other, and where two laws may apply at the same time. This varies significantly depending upon a number of factors including:

- where the person is, e.g. hospital, community, residential care;
- the capacity of the person to give/refuse consent;
- the compliance or resistance of the person to receiving the care/treatment;
- if the care/treatment that is being provided is authorised by the MHA;
- the type of treatment - special rules apply to electro-convulsive therapy and neurosurgery;
- whether the person has made some form of advance decision or refusal;
- the involvement of others with specific legal powers to give or refuse consent to care/treatment on a person's behalf.

The descriptions of the MCA and MHA in the following chapters help explain how to deal with situations involving these variable factors, as do the chapters in Part II. However, we have also produced a decision matrix to help nurses identify where they can, and cannot provide care or treatment, depending upon how these different factors apply, given in the Appendix. The decision matrix includes the following seven tables for quick reference:

1. Capacity, consent and compliance: care and treatment in hospital
2. Capacity, consent and compliance: care and treatment in the community
3. Capacity, consent and compliance: care and treatment in care homes
4. Capacity, consent and compliance: care and treatment under MHA short-term powers

5 Advance decisions to refuse treatment (ADRT), LPAs and court-appointed deputies: care and treatment in hospital
6 ADRTs, LPAs and court-appointed deputies: care and treatment in the community
7 ADRTs, LPAs and court-appointed deputies: care and treatment in care homes.

We would emphasise that these tables in the decision matrix should *not* be used as substitutes for the proper use of the MCA and MHA, taking into account the individual involved and the specific circumstances, and making full use of the Codes of Practice, professional knowledge and experience, and other guidance such as this book. However, in many situations, nurses and other staff do not have the time or the knowledge to go through a lot of written guidance to find out what to do, so these tables are designed to signpost what action can be taken according to the situation and laws that apply, and which specific legal factors staff need to take into account.

The Human Rights Act and the Equality Act

Learning outcomes

This chapter covers:

- The Human Rights Act 1998
- Key Articles: 2, 3, 5, 6 and 8
- The Equality Act 2010
- Implications and challenges for nursing practice

The Human Rights Act 1998

'Human rights' are the basic rights and freedoms that belong to every person. They are based on core principles of dignity, fairness, equality, respect and autonomy. They were first set out by the United Nations in the 1948 Universal Declaration of Human Rights. Since then, there have been many international treaties setting out human rights, for instance, the human rights of children (Convention on the Rights of the Child) and most recently, the human rights of disabled people (the UN Convention on the Rights of Persons with Disabilities). The UK has signed up to, and agreed to be bound by, these Conventions.

The UK is also one of 47 European countries that have agreed to a set of human rights that they will guarantee by law to all the people in their country. These are contained in the European Convention on Human Rights (1952). The European Court of Human Rights was also set up to settle disputes when individuals claimed that the state had deprived them of their human rights. It is a unique system of protection of human rights. The rights are now set out in the UK's Human Rights Act (HRA) 1998 that came into force in 2000. As a result, any individual who considers that the government or a public authority has denied their human rights can seek judgment in the UK courts, and, if they succeed, they will receive compensation (and maybe the law itself will be changed). If they do not succeed in the UK courts, they can take a case to the European Court of Human Rights in Strasbourg and sometimes that court may override the UK court's decision.

In addition, the UK Parliament and the courts must make sure that the laws they make are in accordance with the human rights specified in the HRA, and if they fail to do so, those laws will need to be changed. This has occurred on many occasions, particularly in relation to mental health. For example, it was decided that the Mental Health Act failed to respect patients' human rights because a detained person did not have a say in who should act as their nearest relative – and the MHA had to be changed to allow that. The right to liberty (Article 5 – see Box 1.1) is particularly relevant because it provides rules to regulate and limit when a person can be deprived of their freedom. The Deprivation of Liberty Safeguards (DoLS) were brought into the MCA because the European Court of Human Rights ruled that someone was deprived of their freedom by being kept in hospital without the legal protections in place as required by Article 5 (the 'Bournewood' judgment, see Chapter 4).

The NHS is a public authority under the HRA. As a nurse, when you are caring for or treating an NHS patient, or a private patient on behalf of the NHS, you are acting as a public authority and must comply with the HRA. Private hospitals are public authorities when providing services to NHS-funded patients. The HRA therefore has an impact on the work all nurses do unless they are working in a private clinic with a private patient. The most relevant Articles in the HRA are the following:

- Right to life (Article 2)
- Freedom from torture and inhuman or degrading treatment (Article 3)
- Right to liberty and security of person (Article 5) (see Box 1.1)
- Right to a fair process in courts and tribunals (Article 6)
- Respect for private and family life, home and correspondence (Article 8) (see Box 1.2)
- Freedom of expression (Article 10)
- Freedom from discrimination in the enjoyment of rights (Article 14).

Box 1.1 Article 5: right to liberty

Article 5.1.e is the central provision with respect to people under the MHA or DoLS. It permits 'the lawful detention of persons of unsound mind'. This state must be demonstrated by 'objective medical expertise' and 'the nature or degree of his or her mental disorder must be such as to justify the deprivation of liberty' (Winterwerp v The Netherlands 1979 2 E.H.R.R. 387).

The detention is no longer lawful when the particular mental disorder disappears or ceases to be serious enough to justify the person being deprived of liberty. As a result of this, a detained or DoLS patient's mental state must be kept under clinical review and the person must be discharged from detention if these conditions no longer apply. Otherwise their detention will be illegal. This is the case even if the person is in a maximum security hospital and thought to be dangerous.

Article 5 also guarantees the detained person a right to challenge their detention with a 'speedy' access to a court. What is speedy will be decided on a case-by-case basis because it depends on the circumstances and the medical complexity of the case. A waiting period of 8 weeks before the review of a patient's detention has been judged to be too long.

If a person is detained without the required documentation being completed accurately, it may be a breach of Article 5.

Box 1.2 Article 8: right to private and family life, home and correspondence

This right is very wide-ranging. It protects four broad areas:

- Family life is interpreted broadly. It does not just cover blood or formalised relationships.
- Private life is also interpreted broadly. It covers more than just privacy, also including issues such as personal choices, relationships, physical and mental well-being, access to personal information and participation in community life.
- The right to respect for home is not a right to housing, but a right to respect for the home someone already lives in.
- Correspondence covers all forms of communication including phone calls, letters, faxes, emails, etc.

(*Human Rights in Healthcare: A Framework for Action 2008*)

Other important articles in the HRA

Article 6 makes clear that the procedure in a tribunal must be fair to the detained person, must allow them to be heard, and ensure that the evidence on which the hospital is relying in order to deprive them of liberty is available to them, or their lawyer.

Article 3 sets a minimum standard of care for a person in an institution, and serious neglect of people in care homes or hospital can infringe that. In a recent case a mentally ill man kept for longer than 3 days in a police cell under s.136 of the MHA without adequate medical care won his case against the UK government for breach of Article 3 (MS v UK 24527/08 (2012) ECtHR 804). This was also the result in a case involving a man who was very ill with schizophrenia and who committed suicide in prison. In a case taken successfully by his mother against the UK government, it was held that he had not received adequate medical attention. The European Court of Human Rights noted that the particular vulnerability of mentally ill persons and their inability, in some cases, to complain coherently about how they are being affected by any particular treatment must be taken into account in assessing Article 3, and in this case led to a decision that the Article had been violated (Keenan v. UK [2001] 33 EHRR 913).

Article 2 puts a duty on hospital staff with mental health patients to ensure that the standards for hospital policies, training and practice must be high when there is a 'real and immediate risk of a mental health patient committing suicide' (Savage v South Essex Partnership NHS Foundation Trust 2010 EWHC 865). The UK Supreme Court awarded compensation to the parents of a young woman who was a voluntary patient and killed herself when the psychiatrist negligently allowed her to go home from hospital for the weekend) (Rabone v Pennine Care NHS Foundation Trust (2012) UKSC 2, (2012 v)). This case should lead to more careful risk assessment and potentially to more voluntary patients being detained, if necessary through the application of the holding powers in the MHA.

Issues for nurses

Article 8 is very important in relation to care in hospitals or care homes. There are particular issues you need to be aware of, noting also that detained patients are not in the same position as informal patients because they are not permitted to leave the hospital and, for the time, hospital is deemed their 'home' under Article 8.

- Restricting visiting rights of detained patients unduly and without good cause would breach Article 8.
- The right to privacy and dignity include the proper use of observation panels to bedrooms and female nurses being assigned to close or night-time observation of vulnerable women patients.
- Mixed sex wards are not permitted (although what that means is differently interpreted in some hospitals) and they are seldom encountered now. Nevertheless there can be situations in which vulnerable, and sometimes sexually disinhibited patients are exposed to risk or upset from others and the careful attention of staff is needed to protect their Article 8 privacy right.
- A person's right to privacy may be breached by:
  - searches that are too intrusive;
  - excessive or inappropriate use of restraint;
  - medical records that are not kept private;
  - mail that is unreasonably withheld;
  - personal information that is wrongly revealed.
- Excessive conditions placed on Community Treatment Orders (CTOs) that restrict the family and private life of a service user (e.g. placing a curfew or restricting where they should live) when it is not necessary for their mental health would breach Article 8.

Nurses working with people in private care homes or nursing homes are the responsibility of the NHS or a local authority social services department and are also subject to the HRA. Serious neglect or abuse of those in their care may be a breach of Article 3 and moving them from their home may breach Article 8 (in some circumstances).

Most of the rights and freedoms are not absolute. Some have exceptions to them, others can be overridden where necessary, and they also have to be proportionate, because of community demands or limited resources, and if supported by other laws. For example, detention, care and treatment under the MHA are deemed to be legal under the HRA, providing the MHA is applied correctly, even if it means, for example, interfering in someone's private or family life. Likewise, because of limited resources, health services are not required to provide life-saving treatment in all circumstances, or a treatment simply because someone requests it. However, under no circumstances can anyone be subject to torture, inhuman or degrading treatment.

The MCA, the MHA and DoLS Codes of Practice give considerable detail on issues that impinge on human rights. The right to information is a component of Articles 5, 8 and 10. As a result, the MHA requires that whenever a person is detained, the hospital managers must do their best to ensure that he or she understands the legal position (s.132). The information must be given orally and in writing and must cover all the essential aspects of his or her situation. This applies also to people placed on a CTO.

For detained patients, information goes further than this, and includes steps to ensure that the person understands why he or she is in hospital and they will be engaged in making decisions about themselves during their detention.

Restraint, seclusion and sedation

According to the MHA Code of Practice (15.4), patients with a mental disorder may present risks to themselves or others - hyperactivity, self-harming, physical violence or substance abuse - but they are also very vulnerable to over-reaction from hard-pressed staff when their behaviour needs to be contained. The accepted techniques of physical intervention, rapid tranquillisation and seclusion can be used disproportionately. This may violate the law, including Articles 3 and 8. The MHA Code of Practice seeks to prevent that from happening with clear guidance and by requiring each hospital to have policies in place.

A note of reassurance

Nurses working in the health sector are not expected to be experts on the law and if you practise ethically and respectfully, comply with the MCA or the MHA and their principles, and if you follow the Codes of Practice, you should not be in trouble with the HRA.

United Nations Convention on the Rights of Persons with Disabilities

Nurses should also be aware of the United Nations (UN) Convention on the Rights of Persons with Disabilities (CRPD), which the UK has accepted as a set of standards since 2009. It covers people with mental health problems, and people with dementia and learning disabilities, as well as those with physical disabilities. The aim of the CRPD is to ensure that the HRA is meaningful for people with disabilities and includes:

- the freedom to make one's own choices;
- respect for diversity;
- freedom from violence, exploitation and abuse;
- access to justice and equal recognition before the law;
- the right to live independently and fully participate in society.

The CRPD also emphasises the rights of people with disabilities to have the same access to health, education and employment as people without disabilities.

The Equality Act 2010

The Equality Act (EA) 2010 combines several laws to simplify anti-discrimination legislation and covers the whole of the UK. Under the Equality

Act people are not allowed to discriminate, harass or victimise another person because of (among other things) their age, disability, race, religion and belief, sex or sexual orientation. These features are called 'protected characteristics'.

The Equality Act covers 'direct' discrimination, which means providing less favourable treatment because of a protected characteristic, and 'indirect' discrimination, which means that rules, policies and procedures have a greater negative impact on a person who has a protected characteristic in a way that cannot be justified. So, treating someone less favourably because of something connected with a disability (e.g. not providing information about treatment for a mental disorder to a person with a learning disability, when that information is provided to others, because the person communicates using picture boards) is illegal.

The Equality Act applies to services providing goods and services (which includes health and social care services) and to employers including non-statutory sector organisations (e.g. care homes, private hospitals).

Most of the EA is now in force. However, the provisions prohibiting discrimination on the basis of age when providing goods and services are expected to come into force in October 2012.

The Equality Act applies where someone subject to the MHA or the MCA is treated less favourably under either of those laws because they have a protected characteristic. For example, giving a black person who is detained under the MHA more invasive treatment than a white person who is also detained and who has the same presentation and behaviour, without a clinical justification, would almost certainly contravene the Equality Act.

Further reading on the Equality Act

The Equality and Human Rights Commission provides more information about HRA, EA and CRPD, including a helpline. More details at: www.equalityhumanrights.com. *The Human Rights Act: A Practical Guide for Nurses* by R. Wilkinson and H. Caulfield (2000) is an excellent text.

Reflective activity

The HRA and the EA can seem very abstract when you are working on a busy psychiatric ward or in the community with someone who may be unwell. But when you have a few quiet moments think back to any situations or incidents you witnessed where a service user's rights under the HRA or the EA appeared not to have been respected. Perhaps discuss this with a colleague whom you trust, with these questions in mind:

- What concrete evidence was there of the person's rights not being respected?
- What did you do?
- What would you do if you saw it happening again?

Implications and challenges for nursing practice

Nursing practice should positively promote the HRA, the CRPD and the EA. Nurses should obey the law but, even if they are following the MHA and MCA, they may do something that is not compliant with the HRA and the EA. Dealing with this may appear straightforward because most people would say they agree with the rights and freedoms in the HRA and the EA. It would certainly be very questionable if someone who expressed racist, sexist, ageist, homophobic, disablist or other discriminatory views should be working as a mental health nurse. Likewise, it should be obvious that nurses should not provide care or treatment in an inhuman or degrading way, or breach service users' privacy.

However, people's own personal values and beliefs may mean that some nurses may hold views that others would consider inhumane or discriminatory. As professionals they should leave these views 'at the door' when they come into work, and most nurses do. After all, they would not want to be treated in a discriminatory way if they were a service user. However, the appalling treatment of people with learning disabilities by nursing staff at the Winterbourne View Hospital that was exposed in the BBC's *Panorama* programme in 2011 showed that staff can treat people in degrading and inhuman ways.

The rights and freedoms in the HRA and the EA therefore may not always be upheld by nurses. This is likely to create difficult situations for service users, family carers and other staff who have contact with them. And of course, service users and their families may express discriminatory views or act in ways that jeopardise other people's rights and freedoms, when unwell or well. This may make working with them very uncomfortable but remember that these people do not have professional duty in the way that nurses do to uphold the rights and freedoms of the HRA and the EA.

Organisations should have proper policies and procedures for dealing formally with these situations. But these do not always provide a very helpful process for responding at an informal level in everyday practice. Although there are no simple ways of doing this, Chapter 5 on values-based practice should help.

Reflective activity

Think about your beliefs and values. If you have any negative or strong views about one or more of the groups with 'protected characteristics' in the EA list, could these possibly be seen by others to be discriminatory? How would you work with a colleague or a service user from one of these groups?

What examples of organisational policies and practice can you think of in places where you have worked that uphold or reinforce the rights and freedoms of the HRA and the EA? As a starting point, think of staff training, information on the wards, or examples of providing a flexible service to meet particular needs of a service user arising from a 'protected characteristic'.

Key points: Summary

- The Human Rights Act 1998 describes people's basic right and freedoms.
- Organisations such as the NHS and nurses must ensure their services and practice promote people's human rights.
- Laws like the MCA and the MHA must not conflict with the HRA – where this occurs, the law may need to be changed. Detention, and providing care and treatment without consent are permitted under the HRA but only with specific safeguards.
- The UN Convention on the Rights of Persons with Disabilities describes how the HRA should apply to people with disabilities, including mental illnesses, dementia and learning disabilities.
- The Equality Act 2010 makes it illegal to discriminate against people because of their age, ethnicity, disability or sexual orientation.

2 The Mental Capacity Act 2005

Learning outcomes

This chapter covers:

- The background to the Mental Capacity Act being passed by Parliament and why legislation in this area was necessary
- An overview of all the key elements of the Mental Capacity Act (excluding the Deprivation of Liberty Safeguards, which are covered in Chapter 4)

Introduction

The Mental Capacity Act 2005 (MCA) came into force in England and Wales in 2007. For the first time England and Wales had a clear legal framework covering mental capacity issues.[1]

Mental capacity – the ability to make decisions – is an issue that affects everyone. Anyone might fall ill or have an accident which leaves them unable to make decisions for themselves. As many as 2 million people in England and Wales have an illness, injury or disability that may result in them being unable to make decisions, either temporarily or permanently. This includes people affected by:

- mental illnesses
- dementia
- delirium
- learning disabilities (and some learning difficulties and developmental disabilities such as autism)
- neurological conditions such as brain injuries or other conditions that cause confusion, drowsiness or loss of consciousness
- concussion or coma following an injury
- alcohol and drugs (including prescribed treatments).

A further 6 million people provide care, support and treatment to people who may lack capacity, such as families, friends, and staff working in health and social care.

The MCA was passed by Parliament in 2005. Because it required the establishment of new services, organisations and processes there was a two-year implementation period prior to it coming into force in 2007. Additional legal safeguards called the Deprivation of Liberty Safeguards (DoLS) came into force in 2009 (these are described in Chapter 4). The MCA applies to anyone over the age of 16 (and in some specific situations can apply to people of any age) although some parts of the MCA only apply to people aged 18 and over. It establishes principles, processes and structures to support people to make decisions for themselves wherever possible, and it can also make a decision on behalf of someone who lacks the mental capacity to make it for themselves, due to illness, injury or disability.

The MCA applies to all paid staff involved in dealing with mental capacity issues, including nurses and other health and social care professionals, as well as support workers, care assistants, other non-professionally aligned staff and volunteers. It applies to staff working in the NHS and local authorities, as well as in private and voluntary organisations. It also applies to families and friends caring for relatives who may lack capacity, and anyone undertaking research with people who lack capacity. It creates some specific roles for people supporting someone who lacks capacity.

The MCA can cover virtually any decision for someone who may lack capacity, including major ones about healthcare, a person's property and money, and where someone lives, as well as day-to-day decisions about their everyday care, and even decisions about what someone eats and what they do during the day. It therefore also applies to people working in other organisations and businesses who come into contact with people who may lack capacity such as the police, ambulance staff, housing workers, employers, advice workers, benefit and employment advisors, and staff working in shops, post offices, banks, building societies and even staff working in telesales.

The MCA includes a *Code of Practice* which explains how the Act should be used on an everyday basis.

Reflective activity: MCA key points

- It supports people to make decisions for themselves wherever possible.
- It enables people to plan ahead for a time when they may lack the capacity to make certain decisions.
- It provides ways of making a decision on behalf of someone who lacks the capacity to make the decision for themselves, with appropriate safeguards.

Think about service users you have worked with. Can you identify people you have worked with in the three situations described above?

Background to the Mental Capacity Act

In 2003, the government announced that it planned to publish draft mental capacity legislation. This was the culmination of a long process that can be traced back as far as 1989 when the Law Commission began a consultation on decision-making for people who lacked mental capacity. The consultation resulted in a report published in 1995 recommending legal reform in the shape of a single comprehensive piece of legislation for people who lack mental capacity (Law Commission Consultation Paper No. 231, Mental Incapacity, 1995). The report included a draft mental capacity bill. However, a change in government in 1997 and some resistance to legal reform because of concerns about mental capacity and end-of-life decision-making resulted in several years of delay before draft legislation was published and passed by Parliament.

Why was mental capacity legislation needed?

Before the MCA was passed, the legal processes for dealing with mental capacity issues involved a combination of common law, case law and guidance issued by government and some professional organisations (including the UKCC, the Nursing and Midwifery Council's predecessor). This caused a number of problems:

- Health and social professionals were often confused about how to assess capacity, and what legal authority they had to make decisions on behalf of people who lacked capacity because there was no clear legal framework.
- Individuals with illnesses and disabilities were often assumed to be unable to make decisions because of their diagnosis and having decisions made for them by health and social care professionals when they were able to make the decisions for themselves.
- The views of families and friends of people with disabilities and illnesses were often not asked for, or ignored by health and social care professionals.
- Opportunities for people to plan ahead for a time when they might lack capacity were limited, often ignored, and open to abuse.

For these reasons, mental capacity legislation was widely supported by health and social care organisations, professionals organisations (including the Royal College of Nursing), legal professionals, carers organisations, and organisations representing people with mental capacity issues. The MCA brought together common law, case law, and good practice into one coherent legal framework. Importantly, for health and social care staff, it codified existing good practice rather than creating new and different legal processes that had to be followed.

The Mental Capacity Act 2005

The MCA came into force in England and Wales in October 2007 (although certain parts of it had come into force in April 2007). The Deprivation of Liberty Safeguards (DoLS) came into force in April 2009.

Who does the MCA apply to?

The MCA applies to anyone over the age of 16. In some specific situations it can apply to people of any age (see sections below on the 'Court of Protection' and

'Criminal Offence') although some parts of the MCA only apply to people aged 18 and over (see sections on 'Advance decisions to refuse treatment' and 'Lasting Power of Attorney'). It enables anyone to plan ahead if they have capacity but many of its safeguards and processes apply specifically to people who lack capacity to make a decision because of an illness, injury or disability, as described at the beginning of this chapter.

The MCA also applies to families, friends, neighbours and volunteers who are caring for someone who may lack capacity, or who may have to make decisions on behalf of someone who lacks capacity. In some situations they may have been appointed to undertake a specific role under the MCA. This includes:

- an *attorney*, appointed under a *Lasting Power of Attorney* (LPA);
- a *deputy*, appointed by the *Court of Protection*;
- *a relevant person's representative* for someone subject to DoLS (see Chapter 4).

All these roles are explained in more detail below.

Which staff are affected by the Mental Capacity Act?

The MCA applies to all paid staff involved in dealing with mental capacity issues covered by the MCA. In the mental health sector this includes:

- mental health professionals such as nurses, psychiatrists, psychologists, social workers, occupational therapists, psychotherapists, and counsellors;
- non-professionally aligned staff such as support workers, domiciliary staff, day centre workers, care assistants, staff working in supported housing, paramedics, police, probation officers, and prison officers;
- staff undertaking research with people who may lack capacity to consent to the research;
- staff undertaking specific roles created by the MCA:
  - professional deputy, appointed by the Court of Protection;
  - an Independent Mental Capacity Advocate (IMCA);
  - a best interests assessor (BIA) for someone subject to DoLS (see Chapter 4).

The MCA applies to staff working in the NHS and local authorities as well as staff (and volunteers) working for local and national charities (such as Mind and Rethink), and private sector organisations (such as private hospitals and care homes).

Any paid staff involved in dealing with mental capacity issues must, according to the MCA, 'have regard' to the MCA's Code of Practice, which explains how it should be used in everyday practice (there is a supplementary Code of Practice for DoLS). This means that they must follow the Code of Practice, unless there are good reasons for not doing so.

Unlike the Mental Health Act, most of the MCA does not require specific professionals to carry out key functions or processes – any staff can undertake mental capacity assessments and make decisions (or carry out actions) on behalf of a person who lacks capacity if it is in the person's best interests.

Which decisions does the MCA cover?

The MCA can cover virtually any decision for someone who may lack capacity, including major ones about healthcare, social care, a person's property and money, and where someone lives, as well as day-to-day decisions such as those concerning a person's personal care, what they eat, or what they do during the day. It covers decisions involving people who may lack capacity in hospitals, care homes, supported accommodation, hostels, and community settings, a person's own home or family home, as well as places such as prisons, police stations and ambulances.

Reflective activity: What's an important decision?

Think about all the decisions you made today before coming to work or starting studying:

- Did they include what you wore or what you ate?
- Was it important to you that you made the decisions for yourself?
- Would you have minded someone else making the decision on your behalf?

If you answered 'yes' to all these questions you should understand the importance of being able to make everyday decisions affecting your life, or being involved and consulted about those decisions.

Typical decisions that might arise involving your practice as a nurse include the person:

- giving consent to having psychiatric treatment;
- agreeing to go into hospital or a care home, on an informal basis;
- agreeing to allow you to do a home visit and letting you in to their home;
- agreeing to accept practical help with some aspect of their care;
- making decisions in care reviews (e.g. CPA);
- giving consent for you to contact other people who know the service user to share information with them (e.g. GP, family members, etc.);
- giving consent for you to speak on behalf of the service user to other practitioners, services or organisations to share information with them (e.g. social workers, hospital or care home staff, housing workers, etc.);
- adult safeguarding decisions.

Decisions like these will arise frequently and the MCA does not require the involvement of a particular professional or specialist other than the person requiring the decision to be made, e.g. a nurse needing a service user's consent to have an injection.

In routine situations such as these, you as a nurse should be able to assess a person's capacity to make the decision, and if necessary, decide what is in their best interests if they lack capacity to give consent, in keeping with the processes described in the MCA.

However, if the decision is more complex or has serious implications for the individual, you may wish to seek advice and guidance from colleagues with more expertise or experience in mental capacity issues, or refer the situation to a specialist such as a clinical psychologist or psychiatrist (e.g. an informal patient saying they want to discharge themselves from hospital and you are not sure if they are well enough).

In addition to this you may be asked to advise others about a person's mental capacity. Situations might include being asked for your opinion about whether the person has capacity, or if they lack capacity, what your views are about the person's best interests regarding the situations described above and:

- consent to other forms of psychiatric treatment (e.g. psychological interventions);
- consent to tests, assessments and treatment for physical conditions (e.g. general hospital treatments, dental check-ups, etc.);
- decisions about where the person lives/who they live with;
- adult safeguarding decisions.

However, certain decisions are not covered by the MCA, even if they involve a person who may lack capacity, and these are known as excluded decisions (see below). Decisions covered by the Mental Health Act concerning a person's care and treatment for a mental disorder are *excluded decisions*.

Which decisions are *not* covered by the MCA?

Excluded decisions that are not covered by the MCA, even if they involve a person who may lack capacity, are as follows:

- consent to having sexual relations;
- consent to marriage or civil partnership;
- consent to divorce or dissolution of a civil partnership;
- consent to a child being placed for adoption or to making an adoption order;
- voting;
- decisions concerning the person's compulsory care or treatment authorised under the MHA.

No one can give or refuse consent, or make a decision on behalf of someone who lacks capacity on these issues – this is because they are covered by other laws. However, it is possible that a professional may be asked for their opinion about someone's capacity to make a decision if a situation has arisen involving one of these matters. It also does not prevent action being taken to protect someone from abuse or exploitation.

The MCA also does not change the law relating to murder, manslaughter or assisting suicide.

The MCA and the MHA

If all the following conditions apply to an individual who lacks capacity to make a decision, the Mental Health Act (MHA) should be used, *not* the Mental Capacity Act (including DoLS):

- the decision involves detention, care or treatment that could be authorised under the MHA;
- the person meets the criteria for compulsory detention or treatment provided under the MHA;
- the treatment cannot be given under the MCA (for example, because the person has made a valid and applicable advance decision to refuse the treatment – see section below on 'advance decisions');
- they lack capacity to consent to the detention or treatment and they are showing signs of resisting the detention or treatment or there is evidence (such as information from a family member) to indicate that they would resist if they had capacity (but remember that the MHA does not have a capacity test and can also be used for people who have capacity).

If someone is being detained or treated under the MHA, the MCA still applies to *any* mental capacity issue not covered by the MHA, for example, decisions covering the person's physical healthcare needs, or personal welfare issues.

The MCA does allow restraint to be used in certain circumstances (see section below on 'Actions involving care and treatment'), as well as detaining people in a hospital, nursing or care home, using the *Deprivation of Liberty Safeguards* (see Chapter 4).

Part II of this book covers the relationship between the MCA and MHA in more detail.

What are the key principles of the MCA?

The MCA begins with five core principles which must be followed in any assessment, action or decision involving someone who may lack capacity (Box 2.1).

Box 2.1 The five core principles of the MCA

1. A person must be assumed to have capacity unless it is established that they lack capacity.
2. A person is not to be treated as unable to make a decision unless all practicable (do-able) steps to help them to make the decision have been taken without success (see Box 2.2).
3. A person is not to be treated as unable to make a decision just because they appear to be making an unwise decision.
4. A decision or action that is taken under the MCA for or on behalf of a person who lacks capacity must be done, or made, in their best interests.
5. Decisions or actions taken under the MCA must take into account whether their purpose can be achieved in a way that is less restrictive of the person's rights and freedom of action, providing it is still in their best interests if they lack capacity.

Box 2.2 Examples of supported decision-making

- Giving the person information about the decision in a way they can understand it, e.g. explaining technical medical terms, taking into account someone with reading difficulties, etc.
- If it is a complex or important decision, choosing an appropriate place and time of day, e.g. where the person feels most comfortable, avoiding times when the person may be drowsy because of the effects of medication, etc.
- Taking into account possible cognitive and communication difficulties, sensory impairments, difficulties reading or writing, difficulties understanding and speaking English.
- Involving other people who know the person (e.g. a close family member) to explain the information.
- Using specialist communication where necessary, e.g. Makaton, British Sign Language (BSL), picture cards, etc.
- Asking the person to explain the information back to you to ensure they have understood it.

Do you know of examples from where you have worked where a person has been supported to make a decision using one of these approaches?

Are there other approaches you have seen used?

Reflective activity: unwise decisions

Try and think about decisions you have made which you regretted afterwards, e.g. buying something expensive you didn't need, or saying something to someone that upset them when you hadn't meant to.

- Was it important to you that you made the decision for yourself even though it was a bit unwise?
- Would you have minded someone else making the decision on your behalf, e.g. telling you what you can spend your money on or what you can say?

If you answered 'yes' to these questions, you should understand the importance of being able to make your own decisions affecting your life even if they are unwise ones (hopefully we learn from these!).

It is important to remember that even if you believe that someone has capacity to make a decision, others (e.g. colleagues, family members, etc.) may not, so you may still have to carry out an assessment of capacity to find out for sure. An unwise decision or difficulties in making a decision with support may also indicate a person lacks capacity and an assessment is needed, but in these situations you should always start by assuming the person has capacity.

The next section looks at how these principles apply in practice.

Scenario: Leroy and Jim

What do these principles mean in practice? Let's take a simple example involving Leroy, a nurse, asking Jim, a service user diagnosed with schizophrenia, for his consent to have an anti-psychotic injection. Jim has mild learning difficulties. Jim is *not* subject to compulsory treatment under the MHA but even if he were, good practice requires the same process to be followed before using the MHA to compel Jim to have the injection.

Leroy and Jim: assuming capacity

When Jim comes to the clinic for his injection he is out of breath, anxious, dishevelled and quite agitated. Leroy notices this as it has been an indication of Jim becoming unwell in the past, but Leroy remembers the first principle of the MCA means that he should assume Jim has capacity to make a decision about having the injection.

Leroy and Jim: supported decision-making

Leroy invites Jim into the room where the injection will be given. He asks Jim if he's feeling OK. Jim says that he had to run to catch the bus and is also worried because he lost some money. He says he wouldn't mind a cup of tea but he has lots to do and isn't sure about having the injection today because it makes him feel drowsy. Leroy makes Jim a cup of tea and lets Jim relax. Then Leroy talks to him about the injection. He asks for Jim's consent to be given the injection. Leroy explains that it's Jim's decision to have the injection and tells him why he has been prescribed that treatment. He gives Jim some information about dealing with the side effects. Leroy makes sure that Jim understands what he has told him by asking him questions.

Leroy and Jim: unwise decisions

Jim listens to Leroy and asks him some questions about the side effects. In the end, Jim asks if he can postpone the injection until the following week. Leroy has used the conversation with Jim to come to a conclusion about Jim's mental capacity based upon the two-stage test of capacity (see Box 2.3). Leroy knows that Jim has a diagnosis of schizophrenia and a learning difficulty that may affect his decision-making. However, he decides that Jim is still able to understand, retain, use and weigh up the information to make the decision not to have the injection (see Box 2.3). Leroy thinks that it may be an unwise decision to postpone the injection because there is the possibility that Jim may start to get unwell again but he knows that Jim's care plan allows for some flexibility regarding his treatment. Leroy tells Jim that he understands his reasons and is willing to postpone the injection but emphasises that he would start getting concerned if Jim didn't have his injection the following week. Jim agrees and Leroy records the meeting in Jim's notes, including a brief explanation of his assessment of Jim's mental capacity.

(continued)

Leroy and Jim: assessing capacity

As the example of Leroy and Jim indicates, an assessment of someone's capacity can be done quite informally. In Jim's case, Leroy used his knowledge of Jim together with good communication skills to decide Jim had capacity to refuse the injection. Leroy adhered to the first three principles of the MCA by assuming Jim had capacity, giving him time, and supporting him with good communication and information to make the decision (while at the same time assessing Jim's capacity to make the decision) and concluding it was an unwise decision but this did not mean that Jim lacked capacity.

Box 2.3 The two-stage test of capacity

The MCA sets out a simple, two-stage test to assess a person's capacity to make a decision. The same test must be used whatever the decision. The test involves finding out the answers to the following questions (described in more detail in the Code of Practice)

1 Does the person have 'an impairment or disturbance in the functioning of the mind or brain'?
2 Does the impairment or disturbance mean that the person is unable to make a specific decision when they need to?

The most typical examples of illnesses, injuries and disabilities that may cause this are those described at the beginning of this chapter. If the answer to question 1 is 'yes', then the second stage of the test needs to be carried out.

According to the MCA, a person is unable to make a decision if they cannot do one or more of the following:

- Understand the information that is relevant to the decision.
- Retain that information in their mind long enough to make the decision.
- Use or weigh up that information as part of the decision-making process.
- Communicate, in any way possible, their decision.

Box 2.4 Research indicates . . . supported decision-making

According to the Mental Health Foundation (2012):

- Service users feel that nurses play an important and positive role in shared decision-making processes and helping to make advance decisions about care and treatment for people with mental health problems and dementia.
- Supporting people to make their own decisions and choices, using shared decision-making approaches, and continuing to involve people who lack capacity in best interests decisions are essential parts of nursing practice.

(continued)

For people with learning disabilities this should have been a lifelong feature in their lives but evidence often shows this not to have been the case, sometimes with very negative consequences. It is important that nurses reinforce good practice around decision-making and always take into account the most effective or preferred method of communicating with an individual.

Best interests

If someone lacks capacity to make a decision, then the decision can be made on their behalf. This would normally be done by the person who needed the decision to be made, such as a nurse requesting permission to provide care or treatment to the person lacking capacity. *Decisions made or actions taken on behalf of people who lack capacity must always be done in their best interests*. There are only two exceptions to this (described in more detail below):

- where the person has a valid and applicable advance decision to refuse treatment;
- decisions involving research where the person lacks capacity to consent to participate in the research.

The MCA does not define what 'best interests' are – that's because it will depend upon the person involved and the decision needing to be made. Instead, the MCA lists what must be taken into account when deciding a person's best interests – this is often referred to as the 'best interest checklist'. The checklist is described in Box 2.4 but also includes the factors listed in the section below called 'Other key factors in mental capacity assessments and best interests decisions'. As a nurse, you must consider all the factors listed.

Box 2.5 The best interests checklist

- **Can the decision be delayed?** Assess whether the person may regain capacity and/or if the decision can be delayed, for example, the effect of medication may make people drowsy at certain times of the day, affecting their capacity to make decisions at these times.
- **Encourage participation.** Do whatever is possible to encourage participation in the best interest decisions by the person who lacks capacity – even if they lack capacity to make the decisions, they may still be able to express some views which help inform the best interests decision.
- **Find out the person's views.** What can you find out about the person that gives you an indication of what they would decide if they had capacity, e.g. the person's past and present wishes and feelings, or beliefs and values (religious, cultural, moral or practical)? These may have been expressed verbally to you or to others, or may be written down

(continued)

somewhere – sometimes in things like care plans, crisis plans, crisis cards (often carried by the person), advance statements or directives, sometimes called 'living wills', but not to be confused with 'advance decisions' (see below).

- **Consult others.** Where practical and appropriate, consult with other people who know the person for their views about the person's best interests and if they have information about what the person's views may be. In particular, try to consult:
  - anyone named by the person to be consulted on the decision;
  - family or friends who take an interest in the person's welfare;
  - anyone involved in caring or supporting the person;
  - an attorney appointed under a Lasting Power of Attorney or Enduring Power of Attorney made by the person (see below);
  - a deputy appointed by the Court of Protection to make decisions for the person (see below);
  - an Independent Mental Capacity Advocate (IMCA) *must* be consulted for certain specific decisions, where there is no one else to consult.

Making a best interests decision is *not* the same as 'substitute decision-making' where the decision is based on what you think is the best decision or action to be taken if you were in the same situation.

Now look at the section below called 'Other key factors in mental capacity assessments and best interests decisions'.

Scenario: Alice and Imelda

Let's look at how best interests might work in practice with another example. Alice is 79 and has been diagnosed with depression. She was recently admitted to hospital voluntarily because she was not looking after herself at home, had been getting lost when she went out, and her family was concerned about her. On admission she was diagnosed with delirium caused by a urinary tract infection. Imelda is the ward manager for the ward where Alice is staying. Alice has always liked going for a walk and decides two days after being admitted that she wants to leave the ward to go to the park.

Alice and Imelda: assessing capacity and deciding best interests

Imelda knows that Alice may lack capacity because of her depression and until her delirium has been properly treated, but starts off by assuming Alice has capacity. She talks to Alice about her decision to go for a walk and what it involves, such as how to get to the park. Imelda quickly comes to the conclusion that this is not simply an unwise decision because Alice is still quite confused and is unable to understand or use the information Imelda gives her. Imelda phones Alice's daughter who lives close by and the daughter agrees that Alice is not safe to go out on her own. She does not think that Alice

(continued)

wants to leave hospital and believes that if Alice had capacity, she would agree to be there. Imelda therefore decides that Alice lacks capacity to make the decision and it would not be in her best interests to allow her to leave the ward unaccompanied. Imelda is also aware of the Deprivation of Liberty Safeguards but the hospital does not have a policy of considering DoLS for people like Alice (see Chapter 4).

Alice and Imelda: less restrictive options

In deciding what is in Alice's best interests, Imelda is very aware that going for a walk is important to Alice. She asked the daughter if she might be visiting Alice soon and if she would be willing to accompany Alice for a walk. The daughter agrees to come in later that day and take Alice out. Imelda explains to Alice that she doesn't want Alice to go out alone but that her daughter will take her out later. Alice is a bit upset but Imelda refuses to allow Alice to leave the hospital alone. Instead she encourages Alice to have a walk in the garden that is attached to the ward until her daughter arrives. Alice agrees and this helps cheer her up. While Imelda believes it is in Alice's best interests not to be allowed to leave the ward, she is also aware of the MCA's fifth principle and therefore doesn't want to restrict Alice unnecessarily.

Imelda records in Alice's notes a brief explanation of her assessment of Alice's mental capacity and best interests decision.

Alice and Imelda: deciding best interests (again)

Similar to an assessment of capacity, deciding what is in a person's best interests may be done quite informally. Having established that Alice lacked capacity to make decisions involving going for a walk, Imelda used the best interests 'checklist' to decide what to do. She involved Alice as much as possible, discussed it with her daughter, took into account Alice's wishes, feelings, beliefs and values (represented by Alice's enjoyment of walking) and decided on a course of action that was less restrictive of Alice's freedoms than simply preventing her from going for a walk.

Box 2.6 Research indicates . . . capacity assessments and best interests

A capacity assessment and any best interests decisions that might arise from it should occur in the correct sequence around the same time as each other, but sometimes more complex decisions (e.g. hospital discharge or serious medical treatment) require a series of meetings and conversations involving the person, staff, IMCAs (or non-statutory advocates) and family or close friends.

(Mental Health Foundation 2012)

Other key factors in mental capacity assessments and best interests decisions

Mental capacity assessments and best interests decisions must, according to the MCA, also involve the following elements:

- ***Be decision-specific and time-specific.*** Jim's capacity to make the decision about his injection does not mean that Leroy can make assumptions about Jim's capacity to make other decisions, or a decision in the future to have the injection. Leroy will need to reassess Jim's capacity next time he sees him. Similarly, just because Alice lacks capacity to make decisions about going for a walk does not mean she is unable to make other decisions or that she will be unable to make decisions in the future about going for a walk. Once the delirium has been properly treated, it is very likely that she will regain capacity to make decisions like this.
- ***Not jumping to conclusions because of age, appearance, condition or behaviour.*** Leroy and Imelda know that in the past diagnoses of schizophrenia, a learning difficulty, dementia and depression were often wrongly used as proof of lack of capacity, irrespective of the person's ability to make a particular decision. The first three principles of the MCA are designed to prevent this. The MCA also stresses that a person's age, appearance, condition or behaviour should not be used *alone* to assess someone's capacity or make a best interests decision. While being aware that these may be factors connected with a lack of capacity, Leroy bases his assessment on the test described in the MCA. Similarly, Imelda takes into account Alice's age and condition when deciding her best interests but these are not the only factors she considers.
- ***Involvement of specialists and others who know the person.*** A capacity assessment or best interests decision should normally be carried out by the individual who needs the person to make the decision, e.g. Leroy asking for Jim's consent to provide treatment, or Imelda deciding what is in Alice's best interests. *Neither* require a specialist, such as a psychiatrist or psychologist to be involved, although it may be helpful to do so where the person has a complex condition, or the decision itself is a serious or complex one. For example, if Jim refuses to have the injection the following week, Leroy might ask Jim to wait and see his psychiatrist. The psychiatrist might also assess Jim's capacity. Imelda involved Alice's daughter in deciding what to do in her best interests. Similarly, people such as family, friends or support workers would not normally be responsible for assessing a person's capacity or making best interests decision concerning very serious or complex issues. The best interests checklist emphasises the importance of involving others to help decide and this could include mental capacity specialists (e.g. psychiatrists, clinical psychologists), other staff who know the person, advocates (see the section on IMCAs below) as well as family members and friends involved in the person's care.
- ***Practical and appropriate help.*** The person must be given all practical and appropriate support to make the decision themselves such as involving family, friends or other staff who know the person well, the use of specialists such as a speech and language therapist or psychologist, the use of an interpreter

or signer, communication tools such as picture cards, and a setting or environment that the person feels comfortable in. Leroy took into account Jim's learning disability when discussing Jim's decisions and also gave him time to make the decision. The Code of Practice also emphasises that wherever possible a decision should be delayed until the person is able to make the decision, e.g.

- when they are conscious;
- when they are less distressed, or no longer in a crisis caused by a mental health condition;
- when the side effects of medication, e.g. drowsiness, has worn off;
- when they are not under the influence of alcohol or drugs.

- ***Based upon reasonable belief.*** Deciding whether someone has capacity or not, or what is in a person's best interests, do not require certainty beyond all reasonable doubt because the MCA is civil, not criminal law. Leroy came to the conclusion that Jim had capacity based upon a *reasonable belief* and *balance of probabilities*, which is what the MCA requires. Similarly, it was Imelda's reasonable belief that her decision was in Alice's best interests. Reasonable belief and balance of probabilities are relative to the decision involved and the decision-maker. The reasonable belief required of a family carer making an everyday decision on behalf of a relative would not necessarily need to be the same as Leroy's or Imelda's. For more serious decisions, such as a permanent change in accommodation, then the evidence a professional might need about capacity and best interests would be more substantial.
- ***Record-keeping.*** The MCA does *not* require any particular administrative processes to be followed when assessing capacity or making a best interests decision, such as complying with time limits, formal meetings, or special forms to be completed. Depending upon the urgency of the decision, they should be carried out as near in time to the decision needing to be made. In many cases, as with Alice, an assessment of capacity will take place almost at the same time as a best interests decision. Making a record in the service user's notes of who was involved, when and how it was carried out, and the result is important, especially for more complex or serious decisions, but it is less important for everyday decisions, except where a person's capacity is fluctuating.

Box 2.7 Research indicates ... standardised protocols

Standardised assessment protocols of capacity or best interests decisions may be helpful especially where a more formal procedure is required for the purposes of care or treatment but it should still be personalised to the individual and decision involved. However, the MCA does not require a formal protocol and the most important thing is that staff are familiar with the process of assessing capacity and making best interests decisions as described in the MCA Code of Practice.

(Mental Health Foundation 2012)

Reflective activity

Think about a time when you recently had to make a big decision, for example, about where to live. Imagine that you lacked capacity to make the decision. Go through the best interests checklist and make a list of the factors that would need to be taken into account to make a best interest decision on your behalf. Ask a colleague to do the same and compare your lists.

Actions involving care or treatment

Section 5 of the MCA makes it clear that care or treatment can be given to someone who lacks capacity to consent to it provided it is in their best interests, based upon a reasonable belief. Staff (and family and unpaid carers) involved in providing this care or treatment can do so without fear of liability, providing the MCA has been correctly followed. This means that things like care and treatment that require physical contact, or actions concerning a person's welfare that would normally require a person's consent can still be carried out legally. The types of activity this could involve include:

- carrying out examinations or tests;
- providing treatment, including giving medication;
- taking someone to hospital;
- providing care that involves physical contact;
- making welfare arrangements on behalf of the person;
- going into a person's home to see if they are all right.

The MCA also permits someone to pay for necessary goods (e.g. food, clothes, etc.) or services (utility bills, hairdresser, etc.) on behalf of someone who lacks capacity, providing it is in their best interests. However, this can *only* be done using the person who lacks capacity's money, or any other means of payment they have, if someone has authority under a *Lasting Power of Attorney* or from the *Court of Protection* (see below).

Restraint

If necessary, the person lacking capacity can be restrained in order to provide care and treatment and Section 6 of the MCA provides legal protection for people using restraint provided certain conditions apply. Restraint must only be for the purpose of preventing harm to the person, absolutely necessary, and proportionate to the likelihood and seriousness of that harm. Restraint could include:

- physical restraint;
- sedation, using medication;
- keeping the person in a secure environment;
- close supervision by staff;
- preventing the person from having contact with others.

In the case of Alice, Imelda prevented her from leaving the hospital but because she had correctly followed the MCA, Imelda was protected from liability (e.g. if Alice's daughter had accused her of imprisoning Alice). Imelda used some restraint (i.e. not allowing Alice to leave the hospital) but this was only for the purpose of preventing harm and was proportionate – Imelda encouraged Alice to go out into the garden.

Restraint may therefore be used to *restrict* for a very short period someone's liberty who lacks capacity in order to carry out an action that is in their best interests. Where restraint is necessary in order to provide longer-term care or treatment in a person's best interests who lacks capacity by keeping them in hospital or a care home, then this is likely to be defined as a *deprivation* of the person's liberty under the Human Rights Act. A deprivation of liberty requires additional safeguards – but these may vary depending upon a number of circumstances, including whether the person is in hospital or a care home. Because of case law (where the Court make rulings about specific cases) in this area there are different interpretations of how DoLS apply (see Chapter 4).

Box 2.8 A word about restraint

Section 6 of the MCA only applies to prevent harm to the person who lacks capacity and needs care and treatment. What can be done to prevent a patient with capacity, who is not detained under the MHA, from harming themselves? The duty to protect life under Article 2 of the Human Rights Act and the duty of care under common law both come into play if the person is suicidal (see Chapter 1), and so long as the action is proportionate to the seriousness of the harm, there is likely to be protection at law. There is also, a right at common law, to restrain a patient who is doing or is about to do physical harm to another so long as it is reasonable, that is, no excessive force is used and the reaction is proportionate to the harm (Hale 2010).

Independent Mental Capacity Advocates (IMCAs)

The MCA created a new statutory right to advocacy for people who lack capacity under certain circumstances. IMCA services should be available in every locality, usually provided by a third sector (voluntary) organisation. IMCAs provide an additional safeguard for vulnerable, isolated people who lack capacity to make certain major decisions, as part of the best interests process.

A referral must be made by the decision-maker to an IMCA for any best interests decision (before the decision is made) when:

- the person lacks capacity to make a decision involving:
  - consent to serious medical treatment (except treatment being provided under the MHA) – see Box 2.9;
  - consent to a change in the person's accommodation involving hospital, care home or nursing home;

    - a DoLS standard authorisation and the person has no 'relevant person's representative' (see Chapter 4).
- there is no one that it is appropriate or practical to consult with about the person's best interests (e.g. no family or friends, or they live far away and have no contact), other than the staff involved in the person's care (though an IMCA must not be used simply because staff disagree with the views of family or friends).

Box 2.9 Defining serious medical treatment

The MCA does not define what a serious medical treatment (SMT) is because this will vary depending upon the individual and the situation. It can cover both mental and physical health treatments but not treatment given for a mental disorder under the MHA. However, the Code of Practice gives guidance about how to decide if it is an SMT. This includes when:

- there is a fine balance between the benefits and burdens of the treatment, or choice of treatment;
- where the treatment proposed is likely to do the following:
    - have serious consequences for the patient;
    - cause serious and prolonged pain, distress or side effects;
    - would prolong life for a terminally ill patient or result in potentially adverse consequences, e.g. withholding or withdrawing life-sustaining treatment;
    - have a big impact on the patient's future life choices, e.g. interventions for ovarian/prostate cancer or therapeutic sterilisation.

Electro-convulsive therapy (ECT) would normally be considered an SMT.

Which treatments have you been involved in providing to someone who lacks capacity which you, or the person, would define as 'serious medical treatment'? Who else was there to consult with?

A referral to an IMCA may also be made in the following situations where the person lacks capacity but this is discretionary:

- an adult safeguarding decision where the person is the potential victim or perpetrator of abuse (even when there are other people to consult);
- accommodation reviews for a person living in accommodation (e.g. a care home) arranged by a local authority or the NHS.

A person subject to a standard authorisation under DoLS or their representative also has a right to an IMCA if they request one (see Chapter 4).

Box 2.10 Research indicates . . . IMCAs

Involving IMCAs is a statutory requirement but there is still a lack of awareness and understanding by some health professionals about their role,

(continued)

and confusion with other forms of advocacy. Yet where IMCAs have been involved, this has generally improved the best interests decision-making process, and helped health professionals gain more understanding about the individual involved who lacks capacity. IMCAs should not be used to replace family or close friends simply because professionals disagree with their views.

(Mental Health Foundation 2012)

The IMCA has the right to meet the person and see the person's case notes. The IMCA produces a report about the person's best interests which must be taken into account by the decision-maker. For decisions about serious medical treatment, an IMCA can seek a second opinion from a doctor and can challenge a decision, including an assessment of capacity. IMCAs should have completed standard IMCA training and follow the MCA Code of Practice.

Planning ahead

Planning ahead (1): advance decisions to refuse treatment

The MCA enables people with capacity to specify treatments (for physical or mental illnesses) that they do *not* wish to receive at a time in the future when they may lack the capacity to refuse it. People may have a number of reasons why they do not wish to receive a treatment, such as unpleasant side effects. The MCA calls these 'advance decisions to refuse treatment' and it is important to be aware how they differ from other forms of advance decisions (see Box 2.11).

Box 2.11 Some common definitions: advance decisions

Advance care planning – an advance statement that has been produced collaboratively between a service user and others involved in their care.

Advance decisions to refuse treatment (ADRT) – the legal term used in the MCA for advance refusals of treatment and the only form of advance decision that can be legally binding.

Advance directive – another term commonly used for advance decisions to refuse treatment. But some people may also include preferences or requests for care or treatment in an advance directive.

Advance statement – usually means an advance expression of preferences and requests for care and treatment (but may include advance refusals also).

Crisis card – a form of advance statement that has information on what to do if a person is having an acute psychiatric crisis.

Living will – another term for advance directives.

ADRTs can be verbal, in writing, or recorded in some other way.

An ADRT is legally binding providing:

- *it is valid*;
  - it was made when the person had capacity;
  - no undue pressure was put on the person to make the decision;
- *it is applicable* – it specifically applies to the circumstances and possible treatment that is being considered when the person lacks capacity;
- it has not been overridden by a Lasting Power of Attorney (see section below) made after the advance decision was made, giving the attorney the authority to make decisions about the same treatment;
- the treatment is not being provided compulsorily under the MHA for a person detained in hospital;
- the person who made it was aged 18 or over;
- it is in writing, signed and witnessed if it applies to life-sustaining treatment.

If an ADRT is valid and applicable, it is legally binding and must be followed even if it is not considered to be in the best interests of the person (because it was made by the person when they had capacity – it might be an odd decision but the principle about unwise decision would still apply). An ADRT that is for any illness or condition, physical or mental, that is not being compulsorily given under the MHA therefore must be followed, even if the person is subject to the MHA.

There are no specific forms for ADRTs, nor is there any central register. However, if a person has made an ADRT, it is very helpful if there is a copy on their case notes, if they agree to this.

Box 2.12 Research indicates . . . advance decisions to refuse treatment

Advance decisions (refusals of treatment) and advance decisions (expressions of preferences, wishes and requests) for people with both dementia and 'functional' mental health problems can be very useful in giving the person more control and confidence about care and treatment that might be provided when they lack capacity to consent. Advance decisions and statements can also be very useful in guiding decisions by health and social care professionals. They may also reduce the need for coercive interventions for people lacking capacity in a mental health crisis. However, it is also important to take into account the following:

- It is helpful to provide clear information as early as possible to service users after diagnosis about what advance decisions are, including the different legal status between advance decisions, advance statements, and lasting power of attorney (LPA), and how they apply if someone is also subject to the MHA.
- Where possible, have an ongoing discussion with the person and their family and close friends about what they have included in an advance decision or statement to ensure it continues to reflect their views.

(continued)

- Ensure that other staff involved in a person's care and treatment are aware of the existence of an advance decision or statement if the person has made one.
- Advance decisions and statements written by people with dementia may focus on longer-term aspects of care and treatment as opposed to crisis situations for people with other mental health problems.

(Mental Health Foundation 2012)

Planning ahead (2): lasting power of attorney (LPA)

A person with capacity can make a lasting power of attorney (LPA) whereby they authorise someone else, called the 'attorney' (such as a trusted family member or friend) to make decisions on their behalf. An attorney can only make decisions on the person's behalf if the LPA has been registered with the Office of the Public Guardian (see below). There can be more than one attorney, authorised to make different decisions or to make decisions jointly. The attorney must make the decision according to the best interests principle and checklist in the MCA and should follow the MCA Code of Practice.

There are two types of LPA and people can choose one or both:

- *Personal welfare/health LPA* – this authorises the attorney to make decisions concerning care, treatment or welfare on behalf of the person. The attorney can only make a decision as specified in the LPA, when the person lacks capacity to make the decision for themselves.
- *Property/financial affairs LPA* – this authorises the attorney to make decisions concerning the person's property, possessions or money. The attorney can only make decisions as specified in the LPA but can be authorised to make a decision when the person still has capacity to make the decision, as well as when the person lacks capacity to make the decision for themselves.

Anyone can make an LPA but they must be aged 18 or over. There are specific forms available from the Office of the Public Guardian that need to be completed. These need to be signed by someone stating the person understood what they were doing when they made the LPA and they were not tricked or pressured into making it. There is a financial charge for registering an LPA although some people on low incomes may be exempt from the charge.

The Office of the Public Guardian maintains a register of LPAs which can be checked to see if an attorney is authorised to be making a decision that they say they have the power to make.

LPAs replace the system of enduring powers of attorney (EPA) which existed before the MCA came into force. EPAs only covered decisions involving property and financial affairs. EPAs made before October 2007 are still valid providing they have been registered with the Office of the Public Guardian.

Reflective activity

- Do you have an advance decision to refuse treatment or an LPA?
- If you don't, what kind of LPA might you choose or what kind of treatment might you refuse?
- Who would you authorise to make decisions on your behalf if you had an LPA?
- What decisions would you authorise them to make?

The Court of Protection and Court-appointed deputies

The MCA established a new Court of Protection (which replaces the old Court of Protection) which deals with disputes or complex cases that come under the MCA. This includes rulings on assessments of capacity, best interests decisions, and DoLS. It can make court orders or it can appoint someone called a 'deputy' to make decisions for someone who lacks capacity. In certain situations the Court can make rulings involving people who lack capacity who are under the age of 16.

The Court has regional locations although it deals with a lot of cases on paper without face-to-face hearings. Unlike MHA tribunals, the Court does not automatically review cases involving people who may lack capacity. There is no automatic right to a Court hearing and there is an application process if someone wants the Court to hear a case. Some people have to get the Court's permission to make an application. There are various fees to pay if someone wants the Court to hear a case (although some people may be exempt from these).

Deputies

Deputies are likely to be the most appropriate person, in the eyes of the Court, to make a particular decision, or series of decisions, involving someone who lacks capacity. Deputies could include a family member, or a professional (including legal professionals). The deputy can only make decisions that the Court has authorised them to make. They must follow the best interests principle and checklists and should follow the MCA Code of Practice. Deputies are supervised by the Office of the Public Guardian.

Box 2.13 Overriding ADRTs, LPAs and deputies

Decisions contained in an ADRT, or made by an attorney or deputy, can be overridden if they apply to a treatment that has been authorised under the MHA. This is because other factors (safety of the person or safety of others) are deemed to be more important, and someone who *has* capacity but who is subject to the MHA can have their refusal of treatment overridden.

Box 2.14 Healthcare professionals are not the only decision-makers involved in healthcare

In certain circumstances decisions about care or treatment for someone who lacks capacity may be made legally by people who are not the healthcare professionals and as a nurse you have to respect this. These are:

- when the person has made an advance decision to refuse testaments (ADRT) that relates to the decision;
- an attorney authorised to make healthcare decisions under a personal welfare/health LPA;
- a deputy authorised to make healthcare decisions by the Court of Protection;
- a deputy authorised to make healthcare decisions by the Court of Protection, through a Court order.

Deputies and attorneys may have the power to consent to care and treatment on behalf of the person who lacks capacity. This includes treatment for a mental disorder if it is not being given under the MHA. Standard authorisations for DoLS must also not be inconsistent with an ADRT, or decision by an attorney or deputy. However, they do not have the power to require a type of care or treatment to be given. Deputies, attorneys and ADRTs can all be overridden regarding decisions involving compulsory detention and treatment in hospital that are authorised under the MHA. This is because these decisions do not require the patient's consent in any case, and they may be necessary to prevent harm to the patient or to others. For other care and treatment decisions that are not covered by the MHA (e.g. for a physical illness), then their decision must be followed providing they are authorised to make the decision and it is done in accordance with the other MCA safeguards that apply (e.g. attorneys or deputies using the best interests principle and checklist, or that the ADRT is valid and applicable).

Public Guardian

The MCA creates a new public official called the Public Guardian. This person has specific responsibilities under the MCA which are:

- to manage a register of LPAs and EPAs;
- to supervise court-appointed deputies;
- to send Court of Protection Visitors to visit people who may lack capacity (usually when the person has an attorney appointed under an LPA or deputy);
- to deal with inquiries (including complaints) about attorneys and deputies.

The Public Guardian is supported by the Office of the Public Guardian (OPG) and any inquiry about an LPA, EPA or deputy should be directed to the OPG. The address of the OPG is:

Office of the Public Guardian
PO Box 15118
Birmingham
B16 6GX
Tel: 0300 456 0300 (phone lines open Monday–Friday 9–5
(except Wednesdays 10–5)
Fax: 0870 739 5780
Email: customerservices@publicguardian.gsi.gov.uk

Best interests and end-of-life decisions

Mental health nurses do not often find themselves in situations involving treatment necessary to keep a person alive. The MCA does not change the laws on murder and makes it clear that a best interests decision, or any other action under the MCA, must not be motivated by the desire to end someone's life.

However, decisions that involve providing, withholding or withdrawing life-sustaining treatment are covered by the MCA, including those made as part of a best interests decision. Assessing someone's capacity to make a decision about life-sustaining treatment, and the best interests checklist apply in exactly the same way for these decisions as any other decisions. Mental health nurses should therefore be aware of the following issues that may arise in their practice:

- Remember the first and third principles of the MCA (assuming capacity and respecting unwise decisions). People with suicidal ideation or potentially life-threatening illnesses like anorexia nervosa may well not have the capacity to make a decision about life-sustaining treatment but they should still have their capacity thoroughly assessed – it would be discriminatory to assume that just because they are expressing a wish to die that they must automatically lack capacity. The courts recently upheld a decision by doctors not to treat a woman who had taken an overdose who was brought into hospital conscious and expressing a wish not to be treated. The woman subsequently died. Similarly, it would be wrong to allow other views and values to affect the action taken, e.g. automatically deciding that it's 'just another unwise decision' when a frequent self-harmer injures themselves again.
- Artificial nutrition and hydration (ANH – nasal and stomach 'PEG' feeding) are defined as treatment. For people in the final stages of dementia who are unable to drink or feed themselves evidence indicates that ANH may be inappropriate distressing, and even harmful. Best interests decisions may result in ANH being withheld or withdrawn which will lead to the person dying.
- Advance decisions to refuse treatment (ADRTs) can include decisions to refuse life-sustaining treatment (including ANH) but special conditions apply. These include the ADRT being in writing, including a statement that the ADRT applies even if the person's life is at risk, and it must be signed and witnessed. It is particularly important to establish the validity and applicability of an ADRT concerning life-sustaining treatment – especially the person's mental health when they made it, if, for example, it involves refusal of treatment for self-injury or for anorexia nervosa. However, if valid and

applicable, ADRTs are legally binding and must be followed, even if they are not seen to be in the person's best interests (unless treatment has been authorised under the MHA).

- An attorney acting under an LPA may have been authorised to give or refuse consent about life-sustaining treatment for the person who made the LPA. They must make this decision in the person's best interests and it is possible their decision may differ from professionals who are caring for the person. Any disagreement or dispute may have to be referred to the Court of Protection.
- As a nurse you may be asked to witness an ADRT or confirm that someone understood an LPA they were making. If it involves life-sustaining treatment and you are confident the person understands what they are doing and has capacity at the time they are making it, you could sign it but you might prefer to advise they ask someone else. Whatever you do, you should make a note of it in the person's case notes, inform other staff working with the person, and encourage the person themselves to let others know that they have an ADRT or LPA.

Reflective activity: end-of-life issues

Should people with capacity be allowed to end their own lives? Some believe that people with progressive terminal physical illnesses should be allowed to end their own lives if they have capacity to decide this and the MCA does not prevent this although it is still illegal to assist someone to die. What about people with long-term, severe clinical depression that has proved resistant to treatment who have capacity and express a wish to die? Anorexia nervosa and dementia can both result in death and individuals with those diagnoses may express a wish not to be treated and be allowed to die. Does age make a difference or is this being discriminatory? And if a person has expressed this wish but now lacks capacity, should their wishes still be followed if their families or others involved in their care want to keep them alive? What concerns might disabled people or older people have about these issues?

Research

The MCA has special safeguards for people who may lack capacity to consent to being involved in research (e.g. testing new treatment for people with dementia). If a person lacks capacity to consent to being involved in research, the best interests principle and checklist should not be used to decide if they participate. This is because research, by definition, may involve investigating, testing or evaluating treatments and interventions which might not be successful, and therefore would not be in the best interests of the participant. However, this could still provide important knowledge about the causes, treatment or care of people with a similar illness, condition or disability. It would also be wrong to exclude people who lacked capacity if the focus of the research was on the care and treatment of people with an illness, condition or disability that was a cause of the incapacity.

Instead, the MCA sets out other safeguards for a researcher to decide if someone should participate in a research project including the risks involved, and how invasive or restrictive it might be to the person lacking capacity. The safeguards also include a requirement to consult with someone else such as a family member (but not a professional or paid care worker) for advice about whether the person should take part in the research, and what the person's view would be if they had capacity. If there is no one else to consult, then the researcher can nominate someone – this could be a professional such as a nurse, providing they have no connection with the research project.

If someone who lacks capacity and is a participant in a research project indicates they want to withdraw (for example, if they become upset or distressed), then they must be allowed to withdraw.

Box 2.15 Research indicates ... involving people who lack capacity in research

Deciding whether someone who lacks capacity to consent should participate in research involves a different process to best interests decisions. Evidence shows that professionals and researchers sometimes lack awareness and understanding of this process. In addition to the Code of Practice, there is specific guidance available for researchers from the Department of Health explaining what the MCA says about research (http://webarchive.nationalarchives.gov.uk/+/http://www.dh.gov.uk/en/SocialCare/Deliveringadultsocialcare/MentalCapacity/MentalCapacityAct2005/DH_078789).

(Mental Health Foundation 2012)

Criminal offence

The MCA introduces two new criminal offences: ill treatment and wilful neglect of a person who lacks capacity. The offences can apply to anyone caring for a person lacking capacity including professionals, attorneys, deputies and family carers. For someone to be found guilty of ill treatment they must either:

- have deliberately ill-treated the person, or
- have been reckless in the way they were treating the person.

For someone to be found guilty of wilful neglect, it would usually mean that they deliberately failed to carry out an action involving care for the person that they had a duty to do. Penalties range from a fine to a prison sentence of up to five years.

The Code of Practice

The Code of Practice is a requirement of the MCA, to explain how the law should be followed on a daily basis (Department for Constitutional Affairs 2007). There is a supplementary Code of Practice for the Deprivation of Liberty Safeguards (Department of Health 2008).

The MCA states that certain people must 'have regard' to the Code. This means that they should follow the Code unless there are particular reasons not to – they may have to explain and justify these reasons if required. Other people (e.g. family members) should still follow the principles and processes of the MCA but they do not have a particular duty to follow the Code. People who must have regard to the Code include:

- Anyone who is a professional or is in a paid role who is involved in the care or treatment of a person who may lack capacity – this includes nurses, doctors, social workers, psychologists, OTs, care home staff, and other care staff whether they are working in the NHS, social services, housing, voluntary or private care organisations.
- Attorneys.
- Deputies.
- IMCAs.
- Researchers carrying out research covered by the MCA.

The Code covers in much more detail what this chapter has described. It also includes sections explaining how the MCA relates to other areas. It is not possible to describe in detail these other areas but the following section contains brief summaries:

- *Children and young people* – see Chapter 11.
- *Appointees responsible for social security benefits* – People who are in receipt of social security benefits but who lack capacity to make decisions about managing their money can have someone appointed by the Benefits Agency to do this for them. This might be a close relative or someone in a local authority. The Code makes it clear that the MCA applies to appointees.
- *Adult safeguarding* – Safeguarding is about preventing abuse from happening and dealing with it if it does occur. Local authorities are responsible for adult safeguarding but will do this in collaboration with other agencies including the NHS and the police. Organisations that mental health nurses work for should have safeguarding policies and staff with responsibility and expertise in this area. The MCA Code of Practice includes a chapter on adult safeguarding.

The MCA is itself a safeguarding law because of the protections it gives to people who lack capacity. The MCA should help prevent over-zealous treatment or excessive interference in people's lives (the Human Rights Act also provides protection against these, see Chapter 1). The criminal offence contained in the MCA is a very important safeguard to help ensure that the MCA is used correctly. But sometimes people will have capacity but make unwise decisions which then cause safeguarding concerns. In these situations other safeguarding procedures may need to be used. It may be appropriate to reassess the person's capacity but it is important *not* to decide in advance that the person does lack capacity in order to justify a safeguarding intervention because it is believed that this is in the person's best interests. It is also important to remember that people who have capacity may still require safeguarding, and occasionally, people who lack capacity may abuse other people. If you have safeguarding concerns about an individual you are working with, it is very important to report these to your manager, a colleague with safeguarding responsibilities, or in emergencies, the police.

Settling disagreements without going to the Court of Protection

For disputes and disagreements involving mental capacity issues, an application can be made to ask the Court of Protection to resolve it. However, this is likely to be time-consuming, complex and expensive. Courts and formal legal processes can also be intimidating and confusing for people. The Code emphasises the importance of trying to resolve disputes and disagreements through more informal means of mediation (values-based practice described in Chapter 5 can help with this).

Where informal processes do not resolve disagreements, then formal complaints mechanisms may be the next step. It is important to provide people and their families with information about how they can complain if necessary, and what help they can get to do this (e.g. Patient Advice and Liaison Services – PALS). This may feel difficult if they are complaining about the service you work in, or a colleague, but it is important to remember that as someone with an illness or disability, or as a user of the service, they are likely to have less understanding of how healthcare systems work, in addition to being distressed or in discomfort. These situations are often made worse when people are not treated with respect or taken seriously.

Confidentiality and record keeping

The MCA Code of Practice contains a chapter on these issues but the Act itself does not contain any particular requirements on these issues that affect nursing practice so other laws and organisational policies apply as normal. Decisions about sharing information concerning a person who lacks capacity to consent to this should be done according to what is in the person's best interests and in accordance with the laws on data protection and organisational policies. If the person has an attorney for health and welfare decisions, then they will make the best interests decision about sharing or disclosing information but they must do this in the person's best interests.

Obviously it is very important that mental capacity issues are properly recorded in service user notes. This is particularly the case for mental capacity assessments and best interests decisions where it is crucial, especially for important decisions, that the evidence for an assessment or decision is recorded (including what the decision is about), not just the outcome. 'Mr Smith lacked capacity' or 'we treated Mr Smith in his best interests' would not be sufficient on their own. Where someone is very unwell (e.g. a person with severe dementia in a care home) and lacks capacity to make any decisions most of the time, it may be sufficient just to record the occasions when they can make a decision.

Wherever you work as a nurse, it is important that you are aware of the Code and have access to it when you need to. You can download the Code for free from: http://webarchive.nationalarchives.gov.uk/20110907114137/http://www.justice.gov.uk/guidance/protecting-the-vulnerable/mental-capacity-act/index.htm.

Box 2.16 The MCA and case law

Although the MCA as it stands, together with the Code of Practice, should always be your point of reference it is important to be aware of some key court rulings where the court have made some interpretations of how the law applies in certain situations. Key areas that you need to be aware of where there have been rulings are as follows:

- recognising and taking into account a person's family ties and relationships when making best interests decisions;
- enabling people who lack capacity to live as independently as possible in their own homes as opposed to institutional care wherever possible;
- not using DoLS as a way of confining people for the benefit of services – they are safeguards to protect the person;
- the importance of doing thorough and comprehensive best interests assessments, especially for DoLS authorisations.

Care planning and the MCA

Care planning is a central part of the nursing process in hospitals, care homes and the community. Care planning may vary between organisations and different client groups but the most important type of care planning a mental health nurse is likely to be involved with is the Care Programme Approach (CPA).

CPA is the process of how mental health services assess the needs of a service user, plan ways to meet them and check that they are being met. It is underpinned by a set of principles and values set out in the *Service User Guide to CPA*,[2] which emphasise the collaborative nature of the process:

- Assessing their needs with the service user.
- Developing a plan with the service user, in response to the needs identified and agreed.
- Sharing responsibility with the service user (and others as needed, including family, carers and friends), to put the plan into action.
- Reviewing the plan with the service user and others who provide support, periodically.

The Guide emphasises that all people providing services must do so within a set of personal and/or professional values that value equality, show respect for the services as a person, including recognition of their personal strengths and qualities, respect the views of people who are important to the service user, offer information about reasonable choices the person can expect, and help them feel as in control of the whole process as possible.

In England, most people who are receiving care from specialised mental health services will be on CPA and have had a care coordinator appointed; in Wales, it is expected that all such people will be on CPA. The care coordinator should be in contact with all the services being provided and they keep an eye on how the whole set of arrangements is fitting together. They are a point of contact for the service user, and family carers.

If a person lacks capacity to make decisions about what is included on their care plan, then this should be recorded. The best interests process must be used to decide what is included on a care plan in these situations.

Care plans are also often combined with risk assessments. If someone often lacks capacity to make certain decisions which may put them at risk, then this should be recorded, together with guidance on what should be done if this situation arises. This could indicate what is likely to be in the person's best interests but only if there is very good evidence for including this (e.g. based on previous history). Similarly, if someone has a history of making unwise decisions which put them at risk, this may also be worth recording. However, it is important not to be overly prescriptive because a person's capacity to make a decision where risk is a factor, and deciding their best interests if they lack capacity, should always be done on a decision-specific basis at the time the decision is being made.

Care planning is also discussed in the context of the MHA in Chapters 8 and 9.

Key points: Summary

- Mental capacity means the ability to make decisions. People with mental health problems, learning disabilities, dementia, alcohol and substance misuse problems, and brain injuries may at times have difficulty making decisions.
- Nearly all mental capacity issues for people aged 16 or over are covered by the Mental Capacity Act 2005 (MCA), which came into force in England and Wales in 2007. This includes both everyday and major health and social care decisions.
- The MCA is a legal framework of principles and procedures to support people to make decisions for themselves wherever possible, to assess a person's ability to make a decision, and to enable decisions to be made on a person's behalf in their best interests if they lack capacity to make a decision.
- The MCA makes it clear that a person's ability to make a decision must be judged on a decision-specific basis at the time the decision needs to be made – it does not allow 'blanket' assessments of capacity or best interests decisions to be made on the basis of disability, illness, diagnosis, age, appearance or behaviour.
- Wherever you work as a mental health nurse the MCA will almost certainly apply – but if someone is being detained or treated under the Mental Health Act, then the MCA will not apply to all the decisions made about their care and treatment.
- It is crucial that the person who may lack capacity is kept at the centre of any processes using the MCA, even if they cannot make a decision for themselves, as well as consulting with other people who know the person.

Notes

1 Scotland has its own mental capacity legislation, the Adults with Incapacity (Scotland) Act 2000, which was passed by the Scottish Parliament several years before the MCA. The MCA has some similarities to the Scottish legislation but also significant differences. At the time of writing (2011), the Northern Ireland Assembly was in the process of drafting its own mental capacity legislation.

2 For service users and carers, see Department of Health (2007, p. 5).

3 The revised Mental Health Act 1983

Learning outcomes

This chapter covers:

- Principles underlying the Mental Health Act (MHA)
- The structure and main features of the MHA, including the relevant terminology
- The key concepts and the processes involved in detention through to discharge
- The statutory roles and the main safeguards for patients

This chapter on the MHA is divided into several key sections:

- Introduction – how the MHA affects nurses and the principles and values that you will need to apply
- Statutory roles under the MHA – the functions of professional roles and the roles that nurses may play in the formal processes of detention
- How the MHA works – the formal processes of compulsory powers for civil patients from their admission through to their discharge from the MHA and on to aftercare
- Patients' rights, safeguards and professional duties under the MHA:
  - the rights of the patient to appeal against detention /CTO
  - the role of the advocate and nearest relative
  - the duties of professionals
- Places of safety
- Forensic patients
- Guardianship

In this chapter you will be given a great deal of new information. You might find it useful to make your own list of all the people and bodies who have functions under the MHA as you go through the chapter, and make your own chart as to how they fit into the different stages of the process that a service user goes through – starting from being detained through to being discharged.

Introduction

Most people with a mental illness are treated in the community or in hospital as voluntary patients. Many will not come to the attention of specialist teams but be dealt with through general practice. However, at any time there are about 21,000 people in England and Wales who are detained, or on supervised community treatment under the Mental Health Act (MHA). This figure includes a disproportionate number of men from minority ethnic backgrounds but an equal number of men and women (NHS Information Centre 2011).

The MHA has a different scope and purpose to the Mental Capacity Act (MCA). Whether or not a person has capacity is not relevant as to whether a person should be detained under the MHA or whether other parts of the Act should apply (except in relation to specific treatments). Because the MHA gives powers both to lock people up and to restrict their freedoms, it has similarities with criminal law (although its purpose is not to punish but to protect and to heal). Like criminal law, it contains strict procedures for professionals to follow and important safeguards to protect those people who are treated under it. The MHA also provides for people to be given proper aftercare after they have been discharged, and for the premises where people can be detained to be regularly monitored by the Care Quality Commission (England) and the Health Inspectorate (Wales).

While the MHA provides the structure for the care and treatment of detained patients there are some areas that it does not deal with in any detail. The Code of Practice adds flesh to its bones and must be followed. The Human Rights Act provides a principled framework, the common law fills in the gaps.

Some historical background

There has been law governing people with mental illness since the nineteenth century. From the Lunacy Act of 1890 through to the present day new legislation has been passed (broadly speaking) for every generation. Medical practice has changed, new and more effective treatments have become available and our knowledge about mental illness has developed. These factors and changing social attitudes have all played a part in periodically reshaping the law. Most recently the drivers for change have been human rights and anti-discrimination law, the service user movement and the growth of community services. Some changes occurred because of European Court of Human Rights (ECtHR) judgments which ruled that the MHA contravened the European Convention on Human Rights (for instance, because it did not allow detained patients any say over who should be a nearest relative); others because society demanded a greater voice for patients and their families.

The current Mental Health Act 1983 is thus something of a patchwork. It is based on a 1959 Act that was remodelled in 1983 and it was substantially amended in 2007. These controversial amendments considerably broadened the scope of compulsory powers, added to the powers of professionals and improved safeguards for patients. The revised MHA does the following:

- expands the kinds of professionals, including nurses, who can exercise central functions under the MHA;

- introduces community treatment orders (CTOs) for patients who have previously been detained for treatment in hospital;
- widens the scope of the MHA to include new groups, especially those with a personality disorder;
- introduces more safeguards for patients, including a statutory role for independent mental health advocates;
- improves safeguards for children and young people, including a duty to provide appropriate accommodation for those who are detained.

The revised MHA Code of Practice gives detailed guidance on all aspects of the law and practice and is an indispensable reference for people operating the Act. There has been much commentary on the revised MHA, particularly regarding CTOs, and the Care Quality Commission (CQC) and academic institutions are monitoring the effects of the new law.

Values and principles

The decision whether to use the powers in the MHA involves balancing the person's health or safety (or those of others) with their right to freedom. Well-meaning health professionals can come to different decisions about where the right balance is in any individual case and they may need to explain their decisions before a Tribunal or Hospital Managers' Hearing. For most service users the period of detention is brief, but irrespective of duration they may have found the experience of being compulsory detained distressing, frightening or harmful, even if they feel differently in hindsight.

All these reasons make it all the more vital that staff implementing the Act consider carefully the values they hold, know how to rely on the Guidance, Code of Practice and guiding principles of the MHA and understand where to go for assistance. Whether you work as a nurse in a hospital or in the community, the MHA will affect the way you practise with service users and many other professionals involved.

The Code of Practice

We start any consideration of the MHA with the Principles in the Code of Practice because these must govern every action you take under the MHA. The MHA gives professionals extensive powers and responsibilities over the lives, and care and treatment of service users; accordingly the law is supplemented by a list of Principles in the Code of Practice to guide and to govern the exercise of these powers and responsibilities (Box 3.1).

Box 3.1 The Principles in the MHA Code of Practice

- *Purpose principle*: Decisions under the Act must be taken with a view to minimising the undesirable effects of mental disorder, by maximising the safety and well-being (mental and physical) of patients, promoting their recovery and protecting other people from harm.

(continued)

- *Least restriction principle*: People taking action without a patient's consent must attempt to keep to a minimum the restrictions they impose on the patient's liberty, having regard to the purpose for which the restrictions are imposed.
- *Respect principle*: People taking decisions under the Act must recognise and respect the diverse needs, values and circumstances of each patient, including their race, religion, culture, gender, age, sexual orientation and any disability. They must consider the patient's views, wishes and feelings (whether expressed at the time or in advance), so far as they are reasonably ascertainable, and follow those wishes wherever practicable and consistent with the purpose of the decision. There must be no unlawful discrimination.
- *Participation principle*: Patients must be given the opportunity to be involved, as far as is practicable in the circumstances, in planning, developing and reviewing their own treatment and care to help ensure that it is delivered in a way that is as appropriate and effective for them as possible. The involvement of carers, family members and other people who have an interest in the patient's welfare should be encouraged (unless there are particular reasons to the contrary) and their views taken seriously.
- *Effectiveness, efficiency and equity principle*: People taking decisions under the Act must seek to use the resources available to them and to patients in the most effective, efficient and equitable way, to meet the needs of patients and achieve the purpose for which the decision was taken.

Scenario: Genevieve

Genevieve, aged 38, is an artist who teaches art. She has a diagnosis of bipolar disorder. Genevieve is alienated from her family. She has lived for five years with her boyfriend who has had a good moderating influence on her actions when she is 'high'. At such times she can become sexually disinhibited and has on several occasions taken her clothes off to walk down the main street of the town where she lives.

She has just been found on a roundabout, topless, and wearing heavy make-up, as she says she is being a mermaid. Her boyfriend is on holiday with friends but she is convinced he is not returning– even though he has left his possessions in her flat. She is willing to come into hospital but says she will not take any medication – she hates medication because it affects the chemistry of her body and she prefers to manage her illness her own way. The approved mental health professional (AMHP) and other members of the community team must decide whether or not an application for detention should be made. Genevieve does not necessarily lack capacity to make her

(continued)

own decision about treatment. This would be her second hospital admission. Last time she was an informal patient and she discharged herself after a week. How would you apply the principles of the Act here?

- Would the purpose of the Act be furthered by her detention?
- Could she be effectively treated in the community without compulsion? Would she prefer that?
- Is there a way of treating her with the least restriction?
- Is she able to participate in the decision or is there anyone else who should be consulted?
- What is the best use of resources in this case?

The statutory roles

The MHA creates specific roles for professionals, family members and decision-making bodies. These are as follows:

- *Approved clinician (AC)* – A medical doctor, nurse, psychologist, occupational therapist or social worker who has been appointed as an AC (currently by the strategic health authority). Only a person appointed as an AC can take charge of a detained patient's medical treatment. A patient may have more than one AC involved in his or her care.
- *Responsible clinician (RC)* – An Approved Clinician who has been appointed to take overall charge of the detention of a detained patient or one on a CTO, including powers and duties to grant leave, discharge, etc. The RC has responsibility to keep the patient's situation under review and to discharge him or her if the criteria for detention are no longer satisfied. Hospitals have protocols in place to allocate an RC to the patient.
- *Approved mental health professional (AMHP)* – Usually a social worker but may also be a nurse, occupational therapist or psychologist who has received the required training for the role and been appointed by the local authority. Their role includes making the application for a person to be detained under the MHA.
- *Section 12 approved doctor* – A doctor who has been approved by an Approval Panel as a doctor with special experience in the diagnosis or treatment of mental disorder.
- *Nearest relative (NR)* – A relative of the patient who is appointed by the AMHP in accordance with a list in the MHA and who is given specific roles in relation to the service user.
- *Independent mental health advocate (IMHA)* – A specialist mental health advocate with skills relating to detained patients and whose role is to assist the person while they are detained or a community patient.
- *Second opinion approved doctor (SOAD)* – A psychiatrist who has been appointed to a panel by the Care Quality Commission to provide a second opinion for medical treatment for a patient under the Act.

The responsible clinician

Since 2007, healthcare professionals other than psychiatrists can have a formal role for a detained patient. This flexible system enables the person who is actually in charge of their treatment and knows most about their needs and progress to take legal responsibility for their care.

Therefore, if a psychologist is providing the main treatment in the form of psychological therapies, they would probably have day-to-day responsibility for their care, and the closest therapeutic relationship, so they would be the appropriate RC. However, another Approved Clinician might take a subsidiary role, as a nurse prescriber or a psychiatrist who prescribes medication for the patient.

There must always be an available RC in charge of every detained and community patient at all times, including when the RC is not available or on leave and also if the person changes hospital or moves from hospital into the community. So there must be a system of cover for all situations when the RC is not available.

What role might a nurse play under the MHA?

You may have a formal role as an AC or an RC if you are a first level nurse whose field of practice is mental health or learning disability. To do so, you must complete the required AC training and you must also be able to show that you have the required competencies including knowledge of mental health law and of mental disorders. Once you have become an AC, you are put on a register and you may be selected as the RC for a particular patient. You may also train to become an AMHP.

Other formal responsibilities may include:

- being the prescribing nurse under Part 4 of the Act;
- being consulted by the RC about the renewal of a detention;
- being consulted by the SOAD as to the appropriate medical treatment;
- scrutinising documentation for admission;
- facilitating access of the nearest relative and advocates;
- making a report to a Tribunal, or Hospital Managers' Hearing;
- exercising a nurse's holding powers.

In addition, as a person who is regularly and intimately involved with the service user's care and treatment, you will be well placed to reflect on the service user's progress and their level of risk as well as their views, wishes and concerns. These must be assessed when deciding whether a person should be detained or discharged, as well as all the decisions that need to be made during the period they are under the MHA. You will also need to help the service user understand the law and their rights. There are also a number of legal terms you need to know; these are likely to be referred to in shorthand abbreviations by hospital staff concerned with detained patients. A list of the most common terms is given on p. 74.

How the MHA works

Does the MHA apply to this service user?

If a person is likely to need to be in hospital because of their mental health condition, and if they are resistant to that, or to being treated, they will be assessed to decide whether they should be detained, and, if so, under which section. There are two issues here:

1. Does the person have a mental disorder?
2. Does the person meet the grounds (known as the 'criteria') for detention?

Does the person have a mental disorder? The MHA only applies to people with a mental disorder. This is broader in scope, as a result of amendments in 2007, than previously. A mental disorder is defined in the Act as 'any disorder or disability of the mind' but it needs to be one that is established by 'objective medical expertise'. The best reference guides for what is included are the diagnostic manuals, *International Classification of Diseases* (ICD-10 is the current version) and the *Diagnostic and Statistical Manual* (DSM-IV) but they are only guides.

This new definition proved contentious when the Bill was in Parliament in relation to people with a personality disorder, those with autistic spectrum disorders, child developmental disorders, and paedophiles. Many people representing these groups did not consider they should be subject to detention under the MHA, partly because this was stigmatising for them and partly because it was thought they could not be effectively treated under compulsion. However, the Code of Practice gives an illustrative list of diagnoses, which makes clear that they are included.

However, diagnostic labels do not provide the answer as to whether any particular individual has a mental disorder within the MHA; both a mental state examination and a full clinical history, together with information from the service user wherever possible, and from the family or other carers, will be the essential way in which the professionals will come to their conclusion.

There are some exceptions to the definition (people who are therefore outside the MHA), are the following:

- People who are dependent on alcohol or drugs, but have no other mental disorder. There is no distinction as to the kinds of drugs (people who are actually intoxicated or suffering disorders as part of withdrawal but who are not dependent are unlikely to be covered by this exclusion). However, if a person also has a mental disorder, treatment for the alcohol or drug dependence may be an appropriate part of treating the mental disorder.
- People with a learning disability cannot be detained for treatment, put under guardianship or placed on a community treatment order unless their learning disability is associated with 'abnormally aggressive or seriously irresponsible' behaviour. Otherwise the MHA can only be used to make an assessment (under Section 2).

It is possible for people's mental states to be misunderstood. Erratic or eccentric behaviour or unusual beliefs (especially if seen in someone of a different culture or religion) can be misinterpreted. Stereotypes can also unconsciously influence an assessment.

Scenario: Shirley

Shirley is a 60-year-old woman of African-Caribbean origin. After her husband's death a year ago, she became unhappy and has been seeking to communicate with him through the spirit world but says she is only hearing his ancestors and this causes her great distress. Although previously prudent, she began shopping sprees, for expensive fashion items she never wears. She has reached a financial crisis where her son believes action must be taken before she is bankrupt. He has tried to get her to see a doctor for depression but Shirley refuses, saying she is not depressed, just missing her husband and anxious that he is not 'coming through' from the spirit world.

- Does Shirley have a mental disorder?
- Can you think of stereotyped attitudes towards particular groups of people that may unconsciously influence professionals?
- Which principles should be considered?
- How would they apply in this situation?

Consult the MHA Code of Practice paragraphs 3.5–3.6 to assist you.

Does the person meet the grounds (known as the 'criteria') for detention? Under the MHA, service users may be detained and treated against their will for their mental disorder if they meet the criteria for detention. The person may already be in hospital as an 'informal' patient or they may be brought to the hospital by a family member (usually the person who is their NR) or by an AMHP who may be accompanied by the police. The person might be admitted as an emergency.

The first step will be an assessment of the person to see if they meet the grounds for detention. This may not always be clear particularly if the person is under the influence of alcohol or drugs at the time.

According to Zigmond (2010), the criteria for detention are:

> The person must be, or appear to be, suffering from a mental disorder (or the MHA wouldn't be relevant), that disorder must cause some sort of risk for the patient or other people (or there's no need to intervene), the risk can't be assessed or managed without the person being in hospital (can't detain someone in hospital if they don't need to be in hospital) and the person isn't agreeing to the admission (or they wouldn't need detaining).

A person may be detained either for compulsory assessment under Section 2 of the Act, for emergency assessment under Section 4, or for compulsory treatment under Section 3.

The criteria (for Sections 2 or 3) are:

- the person is suffering from a mental disorder of a *nature or degree* which makes it appropriate for them to receive medical treatment in hospital;
- it is *necessary* for the *health or safety* of the person or for the *protection of other persons* that they should receive such treatment;
- that treatment *cannot be provided unless the patient is detained in hospital*;
- (for Section 3 only) *appropriate medical treatment* is available.

Nature or degree

Whether it is the nature or degree of the patient's mental disorder that leads to the requirement for detention is generally not essential to decide. Generally it is agreed to be both as they are bound up with each other. While the nature of the disorder may link to any history and is associated with symptoms and signs, the degree may also focus on what is happening for them now and the severity of the symptoms.

Scenario: Jane

Jane is a woman with post-natal depression who is managing well with the help of her mental health team until her baby gets bad colic and continuously cries. It so upsets her that her condition deteriorates to the point that she and the baby are both at risk of serious harm. It is the degree of her disorder that makes it important to consider detaining her if she resists any intervention on her behalf.

In hospital

A patient can only be detained under the MHA if they need to be in hospital and the doctors will need to show why that is the case, and why treatment or assessment in the community is not appropriate. The need to be in hospital will relate to the seriousness of their condition and to their safety. Most, but not all such people will lack the capacity to make their own decision about admission.

Appropriate medical treatment

This seems an obvious requirement. Otherwise the person is just being detained as a form of preventive detention to keep them or others safe, which is a contravention of the Human Rights Act. There must be a therapeutic purpose. The MHA says that the purpose of the treatment must be 'to alleviate or prevent a worsening of the disorder or one or more of its symptoms or manifestations'.

It does not need to be the best or ideal treatment in order to be called appropriate but clearly this is not a licence to offer a substandard service. Indeed, the Nursing Code of Practice states that you must provide a high standard of practice and care at all times and deliver care based on the best available evidence or best practice.

Scenario: Ian

Ian is a man diagnosed with a personality disorder and depression who is being treated with medication and cognitive behavioural therapy. However, he is not responding well and, after some consideration, dialectical behavioural therapy (DBT) is proposed as the best alternative, given the strong evidence base for that therapy. There is no DBT therapist available so it is proposed that a psychodynamic therapist works with him instead. There have been promising results for psychodynamic therapy, although the evidence for DBT therapy having positive effects is much stronger.

'Medical treatment' is very broadly defined and includes 'nursing, psychological intervention and specialist mental health habilitation, rehabilitation and care' (Section 145 MHA).

The process for detaining civil patients (Part 2 MHA)

The first decision, if the person is not already in hospital, is to decide under which Section they should be admitted, once it has been decided that they need to be admitted under Section. There are several relevant Sections, depending on the circumstances:

- *Admission for assessment; Section 2 (28 days)*: This is appropriate if there is uncertainty about the nature of the person's illness, what the treatment plan will be or whether the person may agree to treatment at a later stage.
- *Admission for assessment in cases of emergency; Section 4 (72 hours)*: This should be made if it is an absolute emergency, but not because there is just a delay in getting all the opinions for an admission under s.2. It lapses unless followed up by a second medical opinion for an s.2 application.
- *Admission for treatment; Section 3 (6 months)*: The person cannot be admitted under s.3 unless a hospital bed has been identified.
- *Holding application for a patient already in hospital; Section 5 (72 hours)*: This lapses unless followed up by an s.2 or s.3 application.
- *Nurse's holding power; Section 5(4) (6 hours).*

Who has a formal role in the process of detaining a patient?

Doctors always have a role in detaining the patient, AMHPs usually have a role, and ACs and NRs sometimes have a role. The application for detention is made by the AMHP or, occasionally, the person's nearest relative. Even if the NR has taken the initial steps to have their relative admitted, the formal actions are better done by the AMHP who will know the local hospital resources and know the service user from a professional viewpoint. NRs can damage their relationship with their relative, the service user, by taking the formal role. The service user may remain resentful and distrustful of their relative who brought about a situation that they, the service user, strongly opposed.

The AMHP

The AMHP must interview the person and identify their NR. They have to decide:

- whether it is appropriate for the service user to be detained or whether some less restrictive option could be taken;
- whether the treatment available is appropriate.

If the application is for s.2, they must do their best to inform the NR and tell them about their right to prevent the admission and discharge the person. If the application is for s.3, they must consult the NR unless it is not practicable or would involve unreasonable delay. They must make important practical arrangements such as the service user's transport to hospital and care of any children, pets and security of their home.

The medical role

Before the service user can be detained, two doctors, one a 'Section 12 approved' doctor must see the person, interview them and conduct the required medical examination.

Both doctors must be satisfied that the criteria for Section 2 or Section 3 are met. Each signs a certificate to that effect, and if the AMHP agrees that it is appropriate, then the person will be detained under the relevant section.

The emergency process (s.4) is different. The AMHP making the application must have personally seen the person within the last 24 hours. Only one doctor is required for the assessment. Another doctor must examine the patient within 72 hours or the person must be discharged.

If the person is already a patient in hospital, their AC or a doctor may make the application.

Finishing the admission process

All the documentation needs to be properly prepared and lodged with the hospital where the bed has been located but hospitals are not required to accept patients. The patient is formally detained only when the hospital managers accept the papers. Before the service user is accepted, the forms must be scrutinised (and if need be corrected), to ensure the person is not detained illegally. The scrutiny of the documents is delegated to staff members (this may often be a nurse on the ward or medical records).

Once the person has been admitted as a compulsory patient under the MHA, they will be conveyed to hospital (if they are not there already). Then the hospital managers must appoint an RC and a course of medical treatment under the MHA may begin. Part 4 of the MHA has special provisions governing medical treatment.

A nurse's role in the process of detention

A nurse who is able to explain to a distressed and confused service user what is happening and who is able to answer their questions will be of great value. The nurse should follow the NICE (National Institute for Health and Clinical Excellence) Service User Guidelines.

Box 3.2 The NICE Guidelines

The NICE (National Institute for Health and Clinical Excellence) Service User Guideline 136 2011 requires the assessment to be carried out in a calm and considered way.

Respond to the service user's needs and treat them with dignity and, whenever possible, respect their wishes.

Explain to service users, no matter how distressed, why the compulsory detention or treatment is being used. Repeat the explanation if the service user appears not to have understood or is preoccupied or confused. Ask if the service user would like a family member, carer or advocate with them.

The holding powers

The holding powers (s.5) enable a qualified doctor, AC or nurse immediately to prevent an informal patient with a mental disorder from leaving the hospital. The nurse must be a qualified mental health or learning disability nurse and can only exercise the holding power if there is no doctor available. It is done by giving a report to the appropriate officer and the time starts at that point.

The grounds for its use are:

- that the patient is suffering from mental disorder to such a degree that it is necessary for their health or safety, or for the protection of others that they be immediately restrained from leaving hospital; and
- that it is not practicable to secure the immediate attendance of a practitioner (or clinician) for the purpose of furnishing a report.

The patient can be kept for up to 6 hours to await the examination by a doctor for the purposes of an s.2 or s.3 application (if a doctor makes the application, the person can be detained for 72 hours).

Box 3.3 Checklist of what the nurse should consider before exercising the holding power

- the patient's expressed intentions;
- the likelihood of the patient harming themselves or others, or of the patient behaving violently;
- any evidence of disordered thinking;
- the patient's current behaviour and, in particular, any changes in their usual behaviour;
- whether the patient has recently received messages from relatives or friends;

(continued)

- whether the date is one of special significance for the patient (e.g. the anniversary of a bereavement);
- any recent disturbances on the ward;
- any relevant involvement of other patients;
- any history of unpredictability or impulsiveness;
- any formal risk assessments which have been undertaken (specifically looking at previous behaviour);
- any other relevant information from other members of the multi-disciplinary team).

(Code of Practice 12.28)

The decision to invoke the power is the personal decision of the nurse who be instructed to exercise this power by anyone else.

Matters concerning the detained patient

Section 17 leave of absence

A detained patient may ask if they can go home temporarily or the RC may wish to give them leave. This is covered by s.17 of the MHA, which gives the RC the power to give a person formal leave of absence. They can be recalled to hospital at any time in writing by the RC and if they do not return, are classified as absent without leave (AWOL). A person who is AWOL will be searched for and can be returned to the hospital by any of the hospital staff, the AMHP or the police.

What medical treatment can be given?

Under Part 4 of the MHA, medical treatment for mental disorder can be given without the detained patient's consent, although people should always be given the opportunity to consent to their treatment. Part 4 does not apply to all people who are covered by the MHA provisions; those on CTOs or held under short-term powers, such as the holding powers, are excluded.

There are special rules for more invasive treatments, medication after 3 months, ECT, psychosurgery, which apply unless the treatment is urgent. This important topic for nurses is discussed further in Chapter 8.

How long does a detention last?

A patient remains under detention until it lapses, or is renewed, or they are discharged from detention (possibly onto a CTO):

- *Lapse:* An s.2 order expires after 28 days. An s.3 expires after 6 months unless it is renewed for another 6 months. When that time has elapsed it is possible for a Section 3 to be renewed subsequently for a year at a time.

- *Renewal*: The RC may renew a person's detention if the criteria are met. They must examine the patient, and consult at least one person who has been professionally concerned with the patient's treatment and obtain their written agreement that the criteria are met. The second professional must be professionally involved with the patient's treatment and must not belong to the same profession as the RC.
- *Discharge*: This refers to discharge from detention, but not necessarily from hospital. The patient may be discharged in several ways – by the nearest relative, by the RC, by the Hospital managers or by the Tribunal:
  - *discharge by the RC*: The RC must keep the patient under continuous review and discharge them if they no longer meet the criteria for detention.
  - *discharge on to Supervised Community Treatment.* A person on an s.3 order for compulsory treatment can be discharged on to a CTO if they meet the criteria for a CTO and both the RC and the AMHP agree that this is the right course.
  - *discharge by the Hospital Managers or by the Tribunal.* The patient can apply to either body to be discharged from detention on the grounds that they do not meet the criteria for detention. They must be discharged if the criteria are not met.

The Tribunal can discharge a person absolutely; give a deferred discharge, or a conditional discharge for people on a restriction order when medical and social supervision is required.

Reflective activity

Look back at Shirley's case. Let us assume that she is to be assessed for being detained under the MHA. Imagine explaining to her what will happen, i.e. all the formal steps that will occur from the beginning of the process until her discharge, and the time frame that the law lays down for these steps to occur.

Supervised community treatment (SCT)/community treatment orders (CTOs)

Community treatment order (CTO) or supervised community treatment (SCT) – these terms are interchangeable. They cover a person who has been discharged from s.3 or s.37 but has been assessed as requiring some degree of compulsory supervision in the community. They are not technically detained. This is the major reform to mental health practice introduced by the 2007 Mental Health (Amendment) Act.

It is still proving controversial after two years of practice. A central concern is how ethical it is to place restrictions on the freedom and private lives of people who are considered well enough to be living in the community. How effective CTOs are remains to be seen, though they usually involve more service input. Existing research is inconclusive (Churchill et al. 2007).

Box 3.4 How the Code of Practice explains the purpose of CTOs

Supervised community treatment is designed particularly for patients who might otherwise lose contact with services on discharge and subsequently relapse, leading to a cycle of readmissions. They are often called 'revolving door' patients.

The purpose of SCT is to allow suitable patients to be safely treated in the community rather than under detention in hospital, and to provide a way to help prevent relapse and any harm – to the patient or to others – that this might cause. It is intended to help patients to maintain stable mental health outside hospital and to promote recovery.

The power to recall the person to hospital for 72 hours is the essence of the CTO. The MHA says that there must be a sufficiently high risk of harm arising from the patient's illness and it must be sufficiently likely that their health will deteriorate to justify the power to recall the patient to hospital for treatment.

Process of a CTO

The RC makes the decision to put someone on a CTO with the agreement of the AMHP who, according to the MHA, must state in writing that the criteria are met and that it is *appropriate* to make the order. The Tribunal may also recommend that a CTO be considered if it decides not to discharge the patient.

Criteria for a CTO

To be eligible for a CTO the patient must be either on Section 3 or an unrestricted criminal justice order. The criteria are broadly the same as those for detention under these Sections (except that obviously the person must be shown to require treatment in the community not in hospital). There is an additional requirement; it must be necessary that the RC should be able to exercise the power to recall the patient to hospital.

How does the RC decide if a CTO is necessary?

The RC must have regard to the following factors in reaching a judgement:

- the patient's history of mental disorder;
- the increased risk of decline in the patient's health if they were not on SCT;
- any other relevant factors.

Whether or not a person has previously been admitted to hospital, their medical history is relevant.

Box 3.5 What the Code of Practice says on the use of SCT

A tendency to fail to follow a treatment plan or to discontinue medication in the community, making relapse more likely, may suggest a risk justifying use of SCT. Other factors are likely to include 'the patient's current mental state, the patient's insight and attitude to treatment, and the circumstances into which the patient would be discharged'.

Conditions on a CTO

A CTO comes with some conditions that the patient must observe. Patients have to make themselves available for a medical examination - in particular before the Section is renewed. The RC will impose other conditions. The most common ones concern:

- where and when the person should attend for treatment;
- where they should live;
- what behaviours should be avoided (for instance, taking drugs or associating with people who do so).

Conditions may cover any other matters that are 'necessary' or 'appropriate' to the person's mental health but they must be clear, precisely worded so the service user can understand them, and interfere with their freedom as little as possible.

While the AMHP must agree with these conditions before they are imposed, the RC can vary them at any time without any agreement or consultation. There is no right to appeal against them. For instance, the care coordinator may arrange accommodation through the local authority as part of an s.117 care package. In that case there might be a condition that the person remains at that residence.

Medical treatment of CTO patients in the community

When a patient is discharged into the community on a CTO, it will include, as a condition of the CTO, the treatment that the person is to have for their mental disorder. Special rules apply to their treatment. It is a complicated regime, which is important for nurses and will also be discussed in Chapter 9.

Recall to hospital

If a person is recalled to hospital, they can be treated without consent and kept there for up to 72 hours. After that, there are two options:

1. either the patient must be allowed to leave and remain on the CTO;
2. or if they need in-patient treatment, the RC could revoke the CTO, in which case the patient will again be detained under the MHA. The AMHP must agree that this is appropriate.

How long does a CTO last?

The CTO lasts initially for 6 months, can be renewed for another 6 months and thereafter year by year. The person may be discharged from a CTO in the same way as from detention. A CTO is renewed in the same way as a Section 3, namely by the RC after consultation with another professional and with the agreement of the AMHP that this is appropriate.

As with the detention powers, the AMHP, in deciding what is appropriate - whether there should be a CTO and what conditions should be imposed - must take account of social and cultural circumstances and also how they influence the family environment and support structures the service user will have.

Patients' rights, safeguards and professional duties

Challenging a detention: hospital managers

The organisation or individual in charge of the hospital is called the Hospital Manager. They are responsible for detained patients and have specific roles (e.g. checking the validity of detention and CTO papers, referring them to a Tribunal). They hear appeals by patients against their detention, called Hospital Managers' Hearings. Patients can appeal at any time. The hospital appoints a panel of people (who are not lawyers) to carry out these roles. The panel will receive written reports from the RC, the AMHP and a nurse, and if three members of the panel agree, the patient can be discharged. Almost invariably that will be because the panel believes the criteria for detention are not met.

Challenging a detention: the Tribunal

When a service user challenges a detention, they come before a Tribunal. A Tribunal called the First Tier Tribunal (Mental Health) hears applications from patients in England and there is a separate system for Wales. There is an appeal to an Upper Tribunal. The Tribunal is composed of a judge (who presides), a medical member and a lay member who will be a person with expertise and experience of mental health in the voluntary or private sector or the NHS. The medical member must examine the patient personally prior to the hearing.

The patient is permitted to have a lawyer to represent them and family members and advocates may attend. The hearings are held in hospital and usually in private. There is a right to appeal to an Upper Tribunal on a point of law. The process includes the following steps:

- The Tribunal requires reports from the RC, a nurse and an AMHP. These reports should address the criteria for detention in order to assist the Tribunal to decide if the person should be discharged.
- It is up to the detaining authority to establish that the criteria are met, not for the patient to show that they are not met!
- A patient may apply to the Tribunal once in every period of their detention (or after the first 6 months if they are on an s.37), whenever they are put on a CTO, or a CTO is revoked, or if they are subject to guardianship.

- The Tribunal must order the discharge of the patient if the criteria are not met, although they can direct that it be deferred if necessary. With forensic patients who are subject to hospital orders (under Sections 37, 45, 48 or 49), the Tribunal can discharge the person with conditions. This is called conditional discharge.
- If a patient does not apply to the Tribunal - and many do not apply - there are automatic reviews. These were introduced for patients under s.3 who have not had a review within the first 6 months. There is also an automatic Tribunal hearing on revocation of a CTO. Automatic Managers' Hearings are held when a Section is renewed or a CTO is extended after 6 months.

A detailed account of the Hospital Managers' Hearing and the Tribunal hearing is given in Chapter 9.

Aftercare (s.117)

This is the free care a person is entitled to receive from the NHS and local authorities after being detained under the MHA. It covers people on a CTO. The principle behind it is called *the principle of reciprocity*. It means that if a person is detained and treated against their will, there is a reciprocal obligation to that person to make sure they get the health and social care services they need to recover when they leave hospital. The NHS and local authorities have a legal duty to provide this until the person no longer requires it. Accommodation may be one of the services to be arranged.

Before a person is discharged from hospital, there is a 'S117 Meeting'. This is a **care planning meeting** to discuss and decide on the care package required for the person being discharged (see further p. 159).

Nearest relatives

The nearest relative (NR) has a crucial role under the MHA. They may do one of the following:

- apply for the service user to be detained or, conversely, to apply to the Tribunal for their discharge;
- discharge the person directly, subject to giving the RC 72 hours to override their decision with a 'barring order' if the person would 'be likely to act in a manner dangerous to other persons or himself';
- discharge a person from guardianship (this cannot be barred).

Who can be the NR?

They should be someone who knows the service user well and can support them at their time of crisis. The AMHP must appoint the NR when a person is detained. The NR is strictly determined in accordance with a statutory list in the MHA. The spouse or civil partner is the first in line, followed by parents, children, and then more distant relatives. Any of these people living with the person or acting as carer goes to the top of the list. A person who is not a relative but has lived with the person for 5 years can also be an NR, if the person is not married or in a civil partnership. They will be the NR unless there is a relative who is caring for them or also lives with them (the question of who should be the NR in this last situation is quite difficult when the person is living in a residential or group home).

Displacing the NR

Another person can be appointed to NR by the County Court, on an application by the patient, a relative or the AMHP. This will be necessary if there is no NR. Otherwise the listed NR can be displaced on grounds set out in the MHA (s.29) that the NR fulfils the following conditions:

- is incapable of acting;
- unreasonably objects to the making of an application;
- has exercised their power to discharge the patient without due regard to their welfare or the interests of the public or is likely to do so;
- is 'otherwise not a suitable person': for instance, if the AMHP believes that the NR will act unwisely or if the AMHP believes that the patient considers the person unsuitable and would like them replaced. It is up to the court to decide. But any evidence of abuse, or evidence that the service user would be distressed by their involvement, or that the relationship is distant, or has broken down are clear instances of unsuitability.

Scenario: Michael

Michael is 43 and lives alone in London. He has a part-time job and a network of friends he has made through the local church where he is a regular attendee. He was diagnosed with schizophrenia when he was 18 years old but for long periods his health has remained stable. However, he has now become very unwell, and is admitted to hospital for treatment under Section 3. Mary, the AMHP, identifies his mother who lives in Cumbria as his NR but she is too ill to take on the role and would be legally incapable to do so. Mary then asks Michael about any other relatives. Michael tells her that he has a brother who also lives in Cumbria but they do not get on well and have not had contact for many years. Michael does not want him to know about the situation. Still distressed about the possible involvement of his brother, Michael asks to speak with an advocate who advises him to suggest someone else than Mary. Michael is very keen that Sarah, whom he knows from the local church, be appointed. After some discussion Mary approaches Sarah to see if she is willing to act.

Would this be an appropriate case to take to the County Court?

Independent Mental Health Advocate (IMHA)

Advocacy is not interchangeable with giving information and advice. While an advocate does gather information and may show which of a number of alternatives are the most reliable and useful, they do not offer advice on a decision or course of action they think to be in the best interests of the patient.

(National Mental Health Development Unit 2009)

IMHA services exist to give an MHA patient access to independent support from trained experts to get the information they need to understand what is happening to them and around them, what their choices and rights are, and, above all, in getting their voice heard and listened to. The advocate helps the person to become more involved in the process and in decisions about their care and treatment. They help to clarify and communicate the patient's concerns and wishes to the professional staff and to smooth the way generally.

The IMHA is available to a person once they are liable to be detained (this excludes emergency patients), are under guardianship, a CTO, or under the criminal justice provisions of the MHA. They may visit and interview the patient in private, visit and interview the medical staff and (with the patient's consent) view their medical and social service records. The patient may request their services at any time and if not the patient, the NR, RC or AMHP should do so, provided that they see it of benefit.

The IMHA should not be confused with the legal representative who acts for the person in seeking to enforce their legal rights.

Professional duties

The MHA provides a range of supplementary and miscellaneous provisions to protect patients and others.

Hospital managers have a duty to give patients information about IMHAs (s.130D) and their rights under the MHA (s.132) and (s.132D), and to inform NRs of the discharge of the patient (s.133).

There are a number of criminal offences, as follows:

- Forgery or false statements in any document made under the MHA (s.126).
- Ill treatment or wilful neglect of a patient receiving treatment for mental disorder in hospital or home or an outpatient (s.127).
- Assisting a patient or community patient to go absent without leave (s.128).
- Obstructing the inspection of premises, refusal to allow a visit, interview, or examination authorised by the MHA (s.129).

Places of safety

The place of safety is somewhere a person with a mental disorder may be taken if found in a public place and 'in need of immediate care and attention' (s.136). It will generally be a hospital, care home or other care setting, or where necessary, a police station. The person must be examined by a doctor and interviewed by an AMHP with a view to deciding what arrangements to make for their care. The maximum time someone can be held under this power is 72 hours.

Scenario: Joseph

Joseph is aged 29. He has a job with the local council and he lives with his partner, Dave, in a country town. At the age of 14 he experienced a psychotic episode and was diagnosed with schizophrenia. In his early twenties he was detained under the MHA and treated with medication but was severely disabled by side effects and his physical health suffered. He had another admission under the MHA a year later because he had discontinued his medication and became ill. Three years ago he met, and moved in with his partner who has helped him to get part-time work. His physical health and sense of well-being improved and his mental health has remained stable. He recently stopped taking his medication, believing he is now recovered. However, he has just been found slumped in the street. He appears to be hallucinating and to be intoxicated. The police take him to a police station under s.136. As a forensic mental health nurse, Rosie is called to attend. She knows that a police station should only be used as a place of safety on an exceptional basis if the person's behaviour is too disturbed or violent to be assessed in the station; she is also quick to surmise that his condition is not likely to be just extreme intoxication. It is possible to transfer the person to a more suitable place for assessment within the 72 hours and she asks that Joseph is transferred there, as although he initially resisted the police, he is not behaving violently. Joseph has been very scared by what is happening but appears less distressed when the transfer takes place to a mental health suite in a hospital an hour's drive away. Dave is shocked and upset by the incident.

What have you learned about s.136 from this example?

The decision needs to be taken whether to admit him to hospital and, if so, whether under compulsory powers. Which factors from the above information would be relevant to the decision?

The power to enter private premises to remove a person to a place of safety (s.135)

The police also have the power to enter private premises, by force if necessary, to remove a person to a place of safety. This applies if there is someone who is believed to have a mental disorder and is being 'ill-treated, neglected or kept otherwise than under proper control' or someone living alone who is unable to care for himself. This requires a magistrate's warrant, in response to an application from an AMHP. When acting on the warrant, an AMHP and a doctor must accompany the officer and an ambulance should be used. The outcome of this process varies – and does not necessarily lead to an application under the MHA for detention.

Patients concerned in criminal proceedings or under sentence

A large proportion of people who enter the criminal justice system have a mental health problem and, in the prison population, approximately 70 per cent have either a psychosis, a neurosis, a personality disorder, or a substance misuse problem – many prisoners have more than one of these problems.

A person who is before the criminal courts, whether at a magistrate level or in the higher courts, can be *diverted* from the criminal justice system and sent to hospital for compulsory assessment, or assessment and treatment (depending on the Section) under the MHA but only if the offence they have allegedly committed is punishable by imprisonment (this covers most crimes) (see Box 3.6).

The reason for this is that a person whose offence could lead to a prison sentence (if guilty) can also be detained in hospital under the MHA even if they have not been found guilty. The mental disorder need not have contributed to the crime and may in fact have emerged since the crime was committed.

Box 3.6 Definition: diversion

'Diversion' is an important, and humane, part of the justice system for people with a mental disorder. It is a process to ensure that people with mental health problems who enter (or are at risk of entering) the criminal justice system are identified and provided with appropriate mental health services, treatment and any other support they need. Mental health liaison and diversion services provide screening, assessment and onward referral at different stages of the process – often at court. This process is often as an alternative to their undergoing a trial and possibly receiving a conviction, sometimes in order to postpone the trial until they are well enough to participate.

There are different stages at which this might occur under the MHA:

- *When the person is awaiting trial, or during the trial but not available for bail.* They can be remanded by the court to hospital for a report on their mental condition (s.35) or, if the charge is not murder, for treatment (s.36). In the former case, treatment cannot be given without their consent, or alternatively under the MCA. In both cases the court makes its decision on the basis of medical reports.
- *At sentencing, that is, when they have been tried for an offence other than murder.* A court that is passing sentence on an offender who has a mental disorder must obtain a medical report before passing a custodial sentence (s.157 Criminal Justice Act 2003). Under s.37 MHA a court can make a *hospital order* as an alternative to prison if two doctors certify that the person meets the criteria for compulsion (which is usually the case).
- *Under a Restriction order.* An order (under Sections 41, 45A or 49) imposed by the court when they believe that the public may be at a serious risk if the person is either discharged from hospital or sent to a less secure hospital setting

than the one the court has specified. This order has the effect of preventing the RC from acting without the permission of the Ministry of Justice.
- *Under Section 37.* An order by a criminal court that the convicted offender should be sent to hospital rather than to prison. Often this comes with s.41 restriction order.
- *Under Section 48/49.* The person has been remanded in prison awaiting trial and needs hospital assessment and treatment, with an s.49 restriction order.
- *Under Section 47/49.* The person has been found guilty and is in prison but needs to be sent to hospital for assessment and treatment and is sent with an s.49 restriction order.

In some cases it will be found that the person is 'unfit to plead' because they are incapable of following the proceedings or instructing their lawyer because of their mental disorder. A person in prison can also be transferred to hospital if it is deemed necessary when they are in prison or on conditional discharge. Slightly different rules apply at the different stages. No prisoner can be treated compulsorily under Part 4 MHA in prison.

If a person is sectioned under s.37 without a restriction order (this would be appropriate as they are not likely to be considered a danger), they could be discharged, for instance, by their nearest relative making an application to the Tribunal for them to be discharged. The Tribunal might then recommend consideration of a CTO.

Scenario: Shirley: two months later

Two months later Shirley was caught shoplifting three expensive watches, a gold crucifix and six cans of aftershave foam. She says she needs them all. She is aggressive with the store detective when he sends for the police. Among her possessions is a knife which she says is to protect her against 'all those robbers out there'. The store has a policy of prosecuting all offenders and she appears before the Crown Court. She is traumatised by the court but manages to plead guilty. The court is told of two previous offences where she had received a fine and her offence is now imprisonable. In this situation the lawyer might call for psychiatric evidence or the judge call for an independent medical report. She is still denying any mental illness but her daughter wants her to go to hospital for treatment.

What options might the court have for Shirley under the MHA? What issues would arise for the court to consider and what further information might they need?

Guardianship

Guardianship allows a person to receive care outside hospital, but with a degree of supervision from a guardian – the person who is nominated in a guardianship order to provide that supervision. This is used by social services where the person's welfare or the protection of other people requires them to be restricted to some extent. The guardian can decide where the person may live, require them to attend for medical treatment, work, training or education. It is not widely used. The application process also requires an AMHP and two medical practitioners to be satisfied that the criteria are met.

Box 3.7 Checklist of commonly used sections and the terms used to describe them

Section 2 – an admission for compulsory assessment
Section 3 – an admission for compulsory treatment
Section 4 – admission for assessment in cases of emergency
Section 5(2) – application in respect of patient already in hospital
Section 5(4) – holding powers
Section 37 – an order by a criminal court that the convicted offender should be sent to hospital rather than to prison. Often this comes with an s.41 restriction order.
Section 48/49 – the person has been remanded in prison awaiting trial and needs hospital assessment and treatment, with an s.49 restriction order.
Section 47/49 – the person has been found guilty and is in prison but while in prison needs to be sent to hospital for assessment and treatment and is sent with an s.49 restriction order.
Section 17 leave – leave of absence from the hospital granted by the RC.
Section 135 – the power of a police officer to enter private premises to remove a mentally disordered person to a place of safety.
Section 136 – the power of a police officer to take someone in a public place who appears to have a mental disorder and who immediately needs care or control.
Section 117 aftercare – the health and social aftercare which must be provided once a person is discharged from detention.

Transporting and conveying service users

This book does not cover in detail transporting and conveying people between their own homes, hospitals and care homes. This is because nurses are rarely involved in doing this. This is a summary of the key points:

- If the person has capacity, they can only be transported or conveyed with their consent unless they are being treated under the MHA.
- If the person is being treated for a mental disorder under the MHA, then they can be transported or conveyed under the MHA.
- If the person has a mental disorder and meets the relevant criteria, s.135 of the MHA can be used by the police to enter and remove someone from a

private place (e.g. their home), and an s.136 can be used to remove them from a public place and take them to a place of safety.

- If the person lacks capacity to consent to being moved, then it *may* be possible to transport or convey them in their best interests but if any form of restraint is used, it must be done in accordance with s.6 of the MCA.
- DoLS cannot be used to authorise moving someone who lacks capacity to consent to this.

Key points: Summary

- Before a person can be detained, they must meet the definition of mental disorder and the criteria for detention.
- The initial detention is based upon recommendations of medical practitioners. At renewal of the detention, the recommendations are done by two professionals, neither of whom may necessarily be a medical practitioner.
- A person may be detained as an emergency for 72 hours, for assessment for 28 days or for treatment for 6 months.
- People in contact with the criminal justice system may be diverted to hospital at different stages of the criminal process.
- The detention must be kept under review and the patient discharged if the criteria are no longer met.
- The patient may challenge their detention at the Tribunal once in every period of detention.
- A family member, in the role of nearest relative, can play a part in seeking the detention or the discharge of their relative.
- Advocates must be made available to assist the patient when they want them.
- Medical treatment can in most cases be given without the person's consent but in some cases extra safeguards are in place.
- Failure to follow procedures may mean that the detention is illegal and contrary to the HRA.

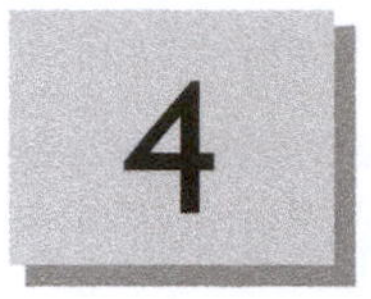

The Deprivation of Liberty Safeguards

Learning outcomes

This chapter covers:

- The background to the Deprivation of Liberty Safeguards (DoLS) being added to the MCA
- An overview of all the key elements of the DoLS and how they relate to the MCA and the MHA
- The changing legal interpretation of DoLS

Introduction

Although the MCA allows restraint to be used under Section 5 (actions in connection to a person's care or treatments), the MCA also places limits on the amount of restraint that can be used. This is because excessive restraint could deprive someone of their liberty under Article 5 (the right to liberty) in the European Convention on Human Rights and the Human Rights Act (HRA) (see Chapter 2).

Restraint could include:

- physical restraint;
- sedation, using medication;
- keeping the person in a secure environment;
- close supervision by staff;
- preventing the person from having contact with others.

At times it may be necessary to restrain someone who lacks capacity in their best interests because they need care or treatment, and this restraint may deprive the person of their liberty. The HRA allows this, providing certain additional legal safeguards are met. The MHA provides these safeguards for people who are detained.

In 2004, a case that was taken to the European Court of Human Rights resulted in a ruling by the Court that identified a gap in the safeguards for people who were detained in hospitals or care homes and lacked capacity to consent to being there but were not subject to the MHA. This gap became known as the 'Bournewood gap' (see Box 4.1) and required extra safeguards being added to the MCA. These are called the *Deprivation of Liberty Safeguards* (*DoLS*). DoLS apply in situations where the restrictions that are placed on a person who lacks capacity amount to a deprivation of liberty and the person is detained in a care home or hospital in their best interests to provide them with care or treatment but the MHA does not apply.

As a nurse it is important you have an awareness and understanding of DoLS as they can affect people with dementia, learning disabilities and mental health problems in hospitals and care homes. As part of someone's care you may have to deprive someone of their liberty and it is crucial that you do this lawfully.

DoLS came into force in 2009 as an amendment to the MCA. There is a supplementary Code of Practice for DoLS which applies in the same way as the MCA Code of Practice (Department of Health 2008). This chapter explains how these safeguards work.

A note of caution is necessary here:

- DoLS may seem very complicated. They certainly look more like legal procedures you would find in the MHA. However, it is important to remember that they are part of the MCA and therefore they should be used with other relevant parts of the MCA (e.g. the five principles, the process for assessing capacity, etc.).
- A large number of cases involving DoLS have gone to the courts and there have been a number of significant rulings by the courts. This means *case law* is particularly important and may not always appear consistent with the Code of Practice. This also means that there are different interpretations of if, how, and when DoLS should be used.

This chapter will indicate where the main differences are, but if you are a practising nurse, you should take advice from your organisation, your colleagues with DoLS expertise, or a lawyer, if you are unsure about a particular situation where DoLS may apply or are being used.

Box 4.1 The Bournewood case

The Bournewood case involved a man with severe autism who lacked capacity to consent to being in hospital but was detained in hospital (called Bournewood Hospital) because doctors believed it to be in his best interests (this happened before the MCA came into force). The man did not resist being detained so he was deemed to be an informal patient and the MHA was not used. The man therefore had no legal protection (such as a clear decision-making process about his detention in hospital, a right to representation, or right for the decision to be reviewed). In 2004, the European Court decided that he had been deprived of his liberty under Article 5 and the UK government therefore had to introduce additional legal safeguards for people in similar situations.

A crucial factor in the Bournewood case was whether or not the man would have given his consent to being in hospital if he had had capacity to make this decision. He did not resist being kept in hospital – had he resisted, and had the other criteria of the MHA applied, then he could have been detained under the MHA. People with severe learning disabilities or severe dementia

(continued)

are rarely detained under the MHA, often because they are not resisting being kept in hospital or a care home, or because other criteria of the MHA do not apply (such as being a risk to self or others, or there being appropriate treatment). DoLS are particularly designed to provide this group with legal safeguards when the MHA does not apply.

DoLS are included in the quick reference tables in the Appendix.

How is a deprivation of liberty (DoL) defined?

The legislation does not define what a DoL is because what counts as a DoL has to be decided on a case-by-case basis. There is guidance for staff to assist them in the DoLS Code of Practice where cases, examples and factors are described. Some examples are given in Box 4.2.

Box 4.2 What might be a DoL?

- Where a service user requires frequent physical restraint or to be in an environment that has been designed to prevent them from leaving the hospital or home.
- Where staff regularly exercise control or close supervision to prevent the service user from leaving the hospital or home.
- Where treatment is used to prevent them from leaving the hospital or home (but if it is *only* being used for this purpose it may not be appropriate use of treatment, e.g. anti-psychotics for some people with dementia).
- Where staff regularly exercise control over who the person has contact with (e.g. family members).

The difference between a DoL and a restriction upon liberty is one of degree or intensity; there is a scale, which moves from 'restraint' (which is defined in the MCA) or 'restriction', to 'deprivation of liberty'. Where any individual is located on the scale will depend on their particular circumstances and may change over time. There may be a combination of interventions which result in a DoL (a 'cumulative effect'). Certainly where the restrictions on someone are unusual or over and above what would normally be required ('excessive' or 'undue' restrictions), then it may well be a DoL.

Situations where DoLS apply

The circumstances under which someone is allowed to be deprived of their liberty are set out in the DoLS provisions which were added to the MCA. In essence, they are as follows (*all* must apply):

- The person has a mental disorder – the definition used is *not* the one in the MCA but the one in the MHA (*'any disorder or disability of the mind'*).

- The person is in a registered hospital or care home – DoLS do not apply to supported accommodation where people have signed their own tenancies, or to people in their own homes (as a tenant or owner occupier). To deprive someone of their liberty who is not in hospital or a care home requires an order from the Court of Protection.
- The person needs to be kept in hospital or a care home to provide care or treatment (for a mental or physical disorder) which is in their best interests (as defined by the MCA) and it may be necessary to protect them from harm.
- The person lacks mental capacity (as defined by the MCA) to consent to the arrangements made for their care or treatment.
- To provide that care or treatment, restrictions must be placed on the person's freedom ('liberty') that exceed the restrictions permitted under Sections 5 and 6 of the MCA (actions in connection with care and treatment) – but see Box 4.3.
- To provide that care or treatment a DoL is needed and is a proportionate response to the need to provide the care or treatment and to likelihood of the person suffering harm and the seriousness of that harm.
- They are not detained under the MHA, or it is not possible to detain them under the MHA because they do not meet the criteria for the MHA – when the person and the situation meet all the criteria for the MHA, then it should be used rather than DoLS. However, where the person is not objecting or resisting, and any care or treatment required is not normally authorised under the MHA then DoLS may apply.
- The proposed DoL, or care or treatment that is to be provided, is not inconsistent with an advance decision to refuse treatment, or the decision of an attorney with an LPA or court-appointed deputy (if they are authorised to make these decisions).

But remember – DoLS do *not* give the power to provide treatment or care (unlike the MHA). It only allows someone to be detained in a hospital or care home. The actual provision of care and treatment must still be carried out in accordance with the MCA. It should only be given with the person's consent (if they have capacity to make the decision) or in accordance with the wider provisions of the MCA, if the person lacks capacity to consent.

Box 4.3 Using the fifth principle of the MCA and Sections 5 and 6

In situations where a DoL for someone who lacks capacity may occur or need to take place, it is also important always to first think about the fifth principle of the MCA – the 'less restrictive' principle. Is it possible to provide the care or treatment that someone needs in their best interests in a way that does not involve a DoL? Can any control or restraint that needs to be used be done just for a short period and/or in a way that the MCA permits without having to use DoLS? It would certainly not be acceptable to continue to use control or restraint required in order to carry out a specific care intervention

(continued)

or treatment after the intervention or treatment had been carried out, nor could this be justified using DoLS.

Sections 5 and 6 of the MCA do permit restrictions to be used on a person if they lack capacity and the care or treatment is in their best interests, and these should be used wherever possible. However, in addition to being proportionate to the risk and seriousness of harm if the care or treatment is not provided, these restrictions are likely to be:

- short-term, e.g. briefly restraining someone who has a needle phobia but needs an injection, or physically guiding someone to a place of safety if they are wandering on a road;
- 'normal' for the care or treatment of people with a similar condition or illness, e.g. having a locked front door in a care home for people with dementia, or physical restraints for people with severe learning disabilities who smear faeces.

DoLS and case law

This is an area where case law is proving to be increasingly important. This is because the courts are hearing a lot of cases in this area and the law is still developing. In deciding what amounts to a DoL the starting point is the concrete situation of the person lacking capacity and that includes all aspects of their life, including whether they are in hospital or a care home. *This may mean that NHS organisations, local authorities, and care homes may interpret the law in different ways and give different guidance or advice – and these may change over time as new case law appears.*

Wherever someone is staying, it is important to remember that DoLS are about a person's human rights – so if you are in doubt or worried about a particular situation, it is essential that good advice is obtained, and if necessary, an assessment for DoLS is carried out. At the same time it is also important to make every effort to avoid DoLS by finding ways to give the person the greatest freedom, consistent with their care and safety – remember the fifth principle of the MCA (always trying to find ways that are less restrictive of a person's rights and freedoms providing they are still in the person's best interests).

Care homes

Residential care homes (see Box 10.1 on p. 169 for a definition of residential care) are generally considered to be a person's home because in most situations it is where the person is permanently living and they have no other home. Restrictions on a person that are deemed to be necessary to provide care and treatment for people in care homes may not amount to a DoL if they go no further than would be required if the person were in their own home (e.g. for their own safety). For example, gently restraining a person with dementia from leaving the home if they lack capacity and it is clear that they need to stay in the home in their best interests. Only if a person was actively resisting, if there were particularly excessive restrictions, or if there was a dispute about the restrictions necessary to keep them in the home to provide the care or treatment (e.g. if a family member was challenging the restrictions) might DoLS be necessary. In these situations it would be important to get the view of the supervisory body (see below).

However, it should *not* be assumed that just because a home used certain restrictions for lots of its residents with dementia that these can be done under the MCA. Again, it would be important to get the advice of the supervisory body.

General hospital

Hospitals are not usually considered to be someone's home. People do not (or should not) 'live' in hospital on a permanent basis. People are not usually detained in general hospital. However, there may be specific situations where someone who lacks capacity to consent to be in general hospital may be detained. The most likely situations are as follows:

- The person is already detained in hospital under the MHA or DoLS for a psychiatric admission and they require treatment for a physical disorder. This can be carried out because the restrictions on their liberty are already in place (though it may be more complicated if they have to be transferred to another hospital).
- The person has been admitted to general hospital for treatment of a physical disorder but lacks capacity to consent to this (but it is in their best interests) and they are resisting being in hospital or the treatment (e.g. a hip replacement for someone with dementia who keeps on getting out of bed to go home). Restrictions that exceed Sections 5 and 6 of the MCA are required to keep them in hospital – DoLS would be required in this situation. If the person was not resisting being in hospital but there was uncertainty about whether they would have consented, or evidence (e.g. from a family member) to indicate that they would not consent to being in hospital, then this may help in deciding if DoLS is required. In these situations it would be important to get the view of the supervisory body.

Psychiatric hospital

Psychiatric hospital is the most complicated area involving DoLS. There has been debate about whether a psychiatric hospital should be considered as home for people who have been detained under the MHA or who lack capacity to consent to being in psychiatric hospital. This is because they cannot freely return to their own home or it is not known if they want to be in their own home. The following list describes the main legal categories for a person's status in a psychiatric hospital and where DoLS may apply (though it would be important to get the view of the supervisory body):

- The person has capacity and gives their consent to being in hospital – they are an 'informal' patient and neither the MCA, DoLS or the MHA applies.
- The person is detained under the MHA (irrespective of whether the person has capacity or not) – DoLS do not apply.
- The person lacks capacity to give their consent to being in hospital and they do not meet the criteria for the MHA but:

  - they are resisting being in hospital ('non-compliant'), e.g. because of the effects of a condition that could not normally be treated under the MHA such as a learning disability, or alcohol or substance misuse - DoLS may apply.
- The person lacks capacity to give their consent to being in hospital and is not resisting being there but needs to be detained to provide care and treatment in their best interests (sometimes referred to as 'non-capacitous, compliant patients'). This is currently the area where it is not yet settled by case law whether this is covered by DoLS. One possible approach is that anyone who is in this category should have DoLS as they would not be allowed to leave, so they must have the same legal protection as patients detained under the MHA. The counter-argument is that it would mean everyone in this situation being detained under DoLS, even those who would have consented had they had capacity.

In situations where the person lacks capacity to give their consent to being in hospital and they do not meet the criteria for the MHA, the pointers in Box 4.4 may help guide a decision about DoLS.

Box 4.4 Indications whether DoLS are necessary

- If there is evidence (e.g. a written statement by the patient, notes in their file, views expressed by a close family member) that a non-capacitous, compliant patient would consent to being in hospital and being treated, then DoLS are probably not necessary.
- If there is evidence that a non-capacitous, compliant patient would *not* consent to being in hospital and being treated, then DoLS (or detention under the MHA) probably are necessary.
- If it is not known whether the patient would consent, then to be on the safe side, an application for DoLS could be made, or at least get the view of the supervisory body.
- If there were particularly excessive restrictions required to keep them in hospital, then DoLS are probably necessary.
- If there was a dispute about the restrictions necessary to keep them in hospital to provide the care or treatment (e.g. if a family member was challenging the restrictions), then it would be important to get the view of the supervisory body about DoLS.

Reflective activity

Think about the last category of people described in the list above – 'non-capacitous, compliant patients'.

- Can you identify people you have worked with who come into this category?
- Was DoLS being used for them?
- Did the hospital give guidance about whether DoLS should be used for them?
- Go back to the example of Alice in Chapter 1 – should DoLS be used?

Compliant or non-compliant?

The quick reference tables in the Appendix refer to the person being 'compliant' or 'non-compliant'. These terms are not used in the DoLS legislation but they are useful to help explain DoLS. Compliant in this context means they do not appear to need any of the interventions, such as those described in Box 4.2, to detain them in hospital or a care home in order to provide them with the care or treatment they need.

A person does not have to be actively resisting to be non-compliant – wandering out of a care home or hospital ward or being removed by relatives when this is not in their best interests could be evidence of non-compliance. If any interventions are considered necessary to detain a person in hospital or a care home, then it suggests that there is the belief that the person may be non-compliant. It is important that there are clear reasons or evidence provided to support this belief.

Procedures

Because they both deal with depriving people of liberty, there are broad similarities between the MHA and DoLS processes and safeguards but also important differences in function and powers.

Unlike the rest of the MCA, DoLS has a formal and quite complicated procedure that must be followed in order for DoLS to be authorised. This covers:

- how an authorisation to deprive someone of their liberty should be applied for, should be assessed, and should be reviewed;
- the requirements that must be fulfilled for an authorisation to be given;
- support and representation required for people who are subject to an authorisation;
- how people can challenge an authorisation.

Statutory roles under DoLS

The DoLS involves certain statutory roles as follows.

Managing authority

The 'managing authority' is any hospital (NHS or private) or care home (with or without nursing care) where a person lives who needs to be deprived of their liberty in order to provide care or treatment that is in their best interests because they lack capacity to consent to this.

The supervisory body

The 'supervisory body' is a local authority in England (or in Wales, the Welsh Ministers or a local health board) which is responsible for considering a deprivation of liberty application received from a managing authority. The supervisory body is responsible for ensuring that the statutory assessments are carried out and, where all the assessments agree a DoL is necessary, authorising it.

Assessors

DoLS requires certain professionals to undertake the assessment of the person in order to decide if the criteria for a DoL are met. There are six assessments (see below) that need carrying out including a best interests assessment. The person doing the best interests assessment is frequently referred to as the *'Best Interests Assessor'* (*BIA*) and is usually a qualified professional such as a social worker, nurse, psychologist or occupational therapist - they can undertake some other parts of the assessment as well (and are often also qualified under the MHA as an Approved Mental Health Professional - AMHP). A suitably qualified doctor must carry out the mental disorder assessment.

Relevant person's representative (RPR)

The RPR's role is to maintain contact with the person, and to represent and support him or her in all the matters that relate to the DoLS, including triggering a review or making an application to the Court of Protection. A close family member or friend can perform this role but it does not need to be the nearest relative, as defined by the MHA. The RPR should be identified at the beginning of the process by the supervisory body. However, the managing authority (i.e. the hospital or care home) must make sure that the RPR understands the DoLS authorisation, and the right of the RPR to request a review and have an IMCA if they want one.

The person themselves may have capacity to say who they want as their representative and if they do this, the person they request should be the RPR. Someone acting as attorney with health and welfare powers authorised by an LPA or a court-appointed deputy for the person might perform the role of RPR or select someone to do this. If none of these are able to select or be the RPR, the best interests assessor will make a choice. The RPR must not be employed in a role related to the person's care or treatment.

IMCAs

A person subject to a standard authorisation under DoLS or their representative also has a right to an independent mental capacity advocate (IMCA) if they request one. A referral *must* be made to an IMCA if the person has no RPR.

The Court of Protection

The Court of Protection can hear appeals against a deprivation of liberty and to order the release of the person if the detention is not lawful.

DoLS authorisations

'Authorisation' is the term used when the supervisory body agrees that someone is being deprived of their liberty and the relevant safeguards are in place. There are two kinds of authorisation:

- *Standard authorisation* – this is an authorisation given by a supervisory body giving lawful authority to deprive a person of their liberty in the relevant hospital or care home.

- *Urgent authorisation* – an urgent authorisation can be given for a short period where the need to deprive the person of liberty is urgent and needs to begin before a request for standard authorisation is given or has been dealt with. It should not be used where it is not expected that a standard authorisation will be needed.

What are the steps involved in getting DoLS for someone?

1. The person is identified as being deprived of their liberty or needing to be deprived of their liberty (this could happen where a person is about to go into hospital or a care home, as part of a care planning process). As a nurse, you may be involved in this process of identification or it may be a family member or another professional who does this. As a nurse you may be involved in actually depriving the person of their liberty if the care or treatment they require is in their best interests.
2. The hospital or care home needs to make an application to the supervisory body. In an emergency, the hospital or care home itself may authorise the deprivation for a maximum of seven days, while the standard deprivation of liberty authorisation process is undertaken – in these circumstances the hospital or care home must reasonably believe that the six qualifying requirements (see point 5 below) for a standard authorisation are likely to be met.
3. The hospital or care home should tell the person's family, and friends and any IMCA or other staff who are already involved, that it has applied for an authorisation of deprivation of liberty.
4. Once the supervisory body receives the application, it must appoint a best interests assessor (BIA) to carry out the best interests assessments (the BIA would normally then contact the other assessor required). The supervisory body should also identify the person's RPR or refer the case to an IMCA straight away if there is nobody appropriate to consult about the person's best interests, other than paid carers or others involved in a professional capacity. This must happen quickly especially if an urgent authorisation has been given because the IMCA is entitled to take part in the process – to receive all the documents that the assessors prepare and to give their views as well as to provide information to the assessors.
5. The assessments are carried out. There are six assessments requiring at least two professionals to see if the person meets all the criteria for deprivation of liberty and to ensure that there is medical and social input into the decision. The assessments cover the following factors:
   - i *the person's age* – (the person must be over 18 for DoLS to apply);
   - ii *the person's mental capacity* – the person must lack capacity to consent to staying in the hospital or care home. This can be carried out by the BIA or medical practitioner.
   - iii *the person's mental disorder* – the person must have a mental disorder as defined by the MHA (not the MCA). This is a medical assessment and must be done by a medical practitioner with the required training. It should usually be a Section 12 approved doctor (a psychiatrist).

  iv *the person's best interests* – the deprivation of liberty is in the person's best interests in order that care or treatment can be provided. This must be carried out by the BIA and must follow the best interests 'checklist' in the MCA.
  v *the person's eligibility* – it is not possible to provide that care under the MHA. This must be done by someone who is an AMHP under the MHA.
  vi *no refusals* – the deprivation must not be in conflict with an advance decision to refuse the treatment that would be provided if the person was deprived of their liberty, or a decision by an attorney acting under a health and welfare LPA or court-appointed deputy who has authority to refuse the decision to deprive the person of their liberty.
6 If the person meets all the criteria and the DoLS is in their best interests, an authorisation can be granted. The BIA must state what the maximum authorisation period should be – this must not exceed 12 months. The underlying principle is that deprivation of liberty should be for the minimum period necessary so, for the maximum 12-month period to apply, the assessor will need to be confident that there is unlikely to be a change in the person's circumstances that would affect the authorisation. An authorisation can come with conditions attached – this might cover such matters as how the DoL should be applied, e.g. who the person can have contact with, when and how he or she can go out, etc. The conditions only apply to the DoL, not the actual care and treatment that is being provided (although sometimes it may be difficult to separate the two).
7 If the person does not meet all the criteria, then an authorisation cannot be given. This is likely to be caused by two main scenarios:
  i The DoL is not in the person's best interests – the care or treatment therefore has to be provided in a way that does not deprive the person of their liberty. The BIA may be able to advise on this but it is likely to require a care planning meeting to work out how to provide the care or treatment the person requires in other ways. If this is not done, the person can take an action for compensation in the courts.
  ii The person does not meet other criteria for DoLS. In this situation the person is being deprived of their liberty unlawfully. Unless other legislation (e.g. the MHA) can be used, the person must no longer be subject to the interventions resulting in their DoL. If this is not done, the person can take an action for compensation in the courts.

Reviewing or challenging DoLS

The person, his or her RPR, an IMCA (if involved) or the hospital or care home itself can request that the supervisory body reviews the authorisation to see if circumstances have changed.

The review should be a formal, fresh look at the person's situation when there has been, or may have been, a change of circumstances that may require a change or termination of a standard deprivation of liberty authorisation. This may occur for example, if a person has regained mental capacity, or the care or treatment that required the deprivation of liberty was no longer needed.

If the result is a decision that the criteria are not met, then the person is immediately released from the authorisation.

The person, or someone acting on their behalf, may appeal to the Court of Protection before an authorisation has been granted or they may appeal once a decision has been reached, to challenge the grounds for depriving the person of liberty, or the length of time or conditions attached to the authorisation.

Scenario: Suzanne

Suzanne is a widow, aged 78. She has been a heavy consumer of alcohol for her adult life and lives in a care home. She has a poor short-term memory, associated with her long-term alcohol consumption and may be a symptom of early dementia.

Her place in the care home is funded by social services. She often goes out for a walk alone to visit her local pub in the afternoons and often returns in an inebriated and distressed state, disturbs other residents by shouting, knocking on doors and sometimes going into other residents' rooms. She has fallen, breaking her wrist once already, after a visit to the pub. She denies that she was inebriated at the time but the staff knew that she had been drinking alcohol heavily that day.

Suzanne lacks any understanding that her alcohol consumption is making her unsafe, and does not accept that it is damaging her health or that she is being disruptive. Her psychiatrist believes that her suspected dementia will advance because of her level of alcohol consumption. Jackie, the senior care home nurse, agrees and is clear that Suzanne does not understand the impact of her alcohol consumption on her health.

The care home staff attempt to get her to drink less, and be less disruptive on her return and they suggest to her son, John, to accompany her at weekends. These interventions have not been effective. Jackie suggests that they might prevent her going out of the care home unless she is escorted – even though this would limit other activities she likes, in particular, chatting in the local shop. Staff escorting her would not allow her to go to the pub. Jackie realises that this may be a deprivation of Suzanne's liberty so she contacts the local authority (the supervisory body). Sarah, a best interests assessor and approved mental health practitioner, undertakes the assessment and John agrees to be Suzanne's RPR. He does not want an IMCA. The assessment is carried out and concludes the following:

- *Age* – Suzanne meets the age criteria.
- *Mental capacity* – It is clear from the assessment of Suzanne's capacity that she is very confused and does not understand the information about the proposed arrangements to prevent her from going to the pub so she lacks capacity to consent.
- *Mental disorder* – Suzanne's psychiatrist confirms that he believes that Suzanne has symptoms of dementia which meet the mental disorder criteria.

(continued)

- *Best interests* – Sarah consults with Jackie, John and Suzanne's psychiatrist about whether the care arrangements are in Suzanne's best interests. Sarah considers the arrangements to be special because of the complexity of dealing with Suzanne's suspected dementia and alcohol problems. She concludes that they are in her best interests.
- *Eligibility* – Suzanne is not eligible for the MHA because the care arrangements could not be provided under the MHA.
- *No refusals* – Suzanne does not have an LPA or court-appointed deputy so there can be no refusals.

Having completed the assessment, Sarah concludes that Suzanne will be deprived of her liberty and that this can be allowed under a standard authorisation which is granted by the supervisory body for six months. The plan includes a requirement for staff to escort Suzanne to the shop twice a week. The psychiatrist also suggested that Suzanne is permitted a small amount of alcohol in the home and Sarah includes this in the plan. John also agrees to visit Suzanne once a week and take her out.

For the first two months the plan seems to work well and staff are able to use appropriate physical restraint (linking arms with Suzanne) to guide her away from the pub, as well as reminding her that she can have a drink back at the care home. However, John is not always able to visit every week. After a couple of months when John does visit, Suzanne keeps telling him how unhappy she is about not being allowed to go to the pub. As a result of this, John believes that the care home is being overly restrictive and too protective. He thinks that Suzanne should be allowed to enjoy herself as she chooses but that she needs to be warned that she will confined for her safety unless she can moderate her behaviour. He therefore requests a review and an IMCA to assist him and his mother.

- What needs to happen next?
- What care issues does this raise if you were Jackie?
- How might it be resolved?

Key points: Summary

- Providing care and treatment in a way that deprives a person of their liberty is a breach of their human rights – this may be the case even if they lack capacity and are not objecting.
- The Deprivation of Liberty Safeguards (DoLS) provide legal safeguards for someone to be deprived of their liberty who lacks capacity and needs to be kept in hospital or a care home in their best interests.
- DoLS are part of the MCA so the principles and procedures such as assessing capacity and making best interests decisions should be followed.

(continued)

- There is no simple definition of what a deprivation of liberty is – it is likely to involve things like restrictions on where the person can go, what they can do, or who the person can have contact with, but each case must be assessed according to the individual circumstances of the person involved.
- You may not need to use DoLS because the MCA allows restrictions to be used with a person who lacks capacity if they are in the person's best interests. This may also be less restrictive of a person's rights and freedoms. But it is important to understand where these restrictions may become a deprivation of liberty and ensure that a person's rights are safeguarded in these situations.
- The MHA also allows someone to be deprived of their liberty and if a person meets the criteria for the MHA, it should be used before DoLS.
- There is a very specific procedure that must be followed for DoLS with particular roles and assessments.
- The law on DoLS is still developing and it is important to seek advice if you are unsure if DoLS are required.

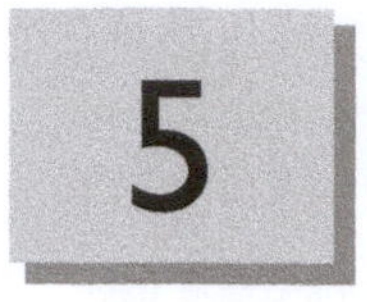

Nursing ethics and values-based practice

Learning outcomes

This chapter covers:

- The importance of values, ethics and principles underpinning mental health nursing in relation to the MHA and the MCA
- The benefits of values-based practice in dealing with tensions and conflicts that arise in mental health nursing in relation to the MHA and the MCA

Introduction

As a mental health nurse it is essential that you do not break the law when caring for people. But as well as ensuring that your practice is *legal*, it is also important to ensure that your practice is *ethical*. The two are not necessarily the same (although it would not be ethical to break the law). Although both are based upon values that guide actions, the law is very specific, whereas ethics are more general principles of professional behaviour. Making sure your practice is legal is necessary but not sufficient ethically; the law does not require you, for example, to care for people in a sensitive and respectful way. Having an understanding of ethics and values in nursing practice goes hand in hand with understanding the law, and is vital in ensuring that service users receive *good* care, not just *legal* care.

Mental health nursing has fundamental differences to other types of nursing, especially in terms of the law. Both the Mental Health Act (MHA) and the Mental Capacity Act (MCA) allow a person to be detained, supervised and treated without their consent. No other major area of healthcare involves legal powers like these.

As a mental health nurse, you know that some people may be so unwell or lacking mental capacity because of illness or disability that they will be unwilling or unable to give their consent to care and treatment that they clearly need. But sometimes there may also be different reasons for thinking that the person may not need the care or treatment – and many people with mental health problems firmly believe that they do not need to be detained and/or treated against their wishes. People may not understand or believe that they have a mental health problem or condition (such as dementia) and may have other reasons for explaining their beliefs and actions.

In other words, people's views and subjective experience of their illness, disability or condition may be very different to those of a nurse involved in their care or treatment. There may be very important differences in the *values* underpinning the beliefs and actions of the various individuals, including professionals, and processes involved when the law is being used. This makes mental health nursing significantly different to nursing people with physical health problems. This can be viewed as a positive asset for mental health nurses because it means the process of decision-making and caring for people is potentially a more inclusive, holistic process, by incorporating a range of different values (including those underpinning the law) and points of views including service users, family carers and other practitioners.

In addition to the values held by individuals and practitioners there are other sources of values, such as codes of conduct and organisational policies that need to be taken into account and followed by mental health nurses and other staff. In situations where the MHA or the MCA may need to be used to compel someone to receive care or treatment, simply following the letter of the law like an instruction manual is not good enough, in the same way that being purely task-focused without taking into account the person you are caring for is insufficient to meet standards of good nursing practice. This is why good nursing practice and the law must intersect with a practical understanding of ethics and values.

The chapters in Part II of this handbook explain how the MHA and the MCA apply in different areas of nursing practice. Each chapter includes references to ethical and 'values-based' practice to help you deal with some of the difficult dilemmas and conflicts that the MHA and the MCA may generate when applied to people you are working with, and in different situations. This chapter explains the importance of ethics and values in mental health nursing and describes the model of *values-based practice* in relation to the MHA and the MCA. For these reasons it is essential that you read this chapter.

Ethics and values in mental health nursing

As a mental health nurse it is essential that you practise according to the law. This handbook has been written to help you do that. But you must also practise in accordance with your clinical training and expertise, together with organisational policies and procedures and with the nursing and midwifery code of professional conduct (NMC 2008). And of course, you must as far as possible follow and respect the wishes and feelings of service users, the views of their families, and other professionals and staff. All of these people and elements to your practice have, or contain, values.

Documents like the NMC code of conduct, or the codes of practice for the MHA and the MCA explain how you put the values contained within them into practice – in other words, how you practise *ethically*. But as we shall see, different people, policies, codes and professional practice in mental health nursing especially, often involve situations where there are competing values – where values are in tension with each other, or in direct conflict. This certainly includes situations where the MCA or the MHA may need to be used to compel someone to receive care or treatment. This can be challenging and difficult to deal with, particularly when you may not have much time, or resources are not always available. But it also makes working in mental health immensely rewarding when you get it right.

Definitions

So what are ethics and values? Ethics and values may sometimes seem complex or irrelevant to everyday nursing practice. It is true that they can be discussed in great detail in philosophical debates which may not be very relevant, connecting with other concepts such as principles, morals and beliefs. But as this chapter will show, it is very important to have a basic grasp of what they mean, and the ways in which they definitely *are* relevant to your practice as a mental health nurse. It's worth starting off by considering the definitions in Box 5.1.

Box 5.1 Definitions

- *Values* – principles you have which control your behaviour – or words guiding actions and decisions.
- *Ethics* – systems of accepted beliefs which control behaviour, especially a system based on morals.
- *Principles* – moral rules or standards of good behaviour.
- *Morals* – standards of good or bad behaviour, fairness, respect, etc. which each person believes in, rather than laws or other standards.
- *Beliefs* – feelings of certainty that something exists or is true.

Reflective activity

- Think of some examples of where these values and beliefs appear in your nursing practice.
- Think of some examples of these in your personal life.
- Are there examples that appear in both your personal and professional life?

Ethics, principles and values

Nursing has a strong ethical base, underpinned by ethical theory. There are two main ethical theories used to guide and justify actions:

- *Deontological theories* – These are concerned with 'duty' or universal rules which should be applied in any situations. For example, intervening to try and prevent someone from committing suicide is an action that most people would consider to be a good thing and is based upon these kinds of theories.

- *Consequentialist (teleogical) theories* – These are concerned with the consequences of actions, i.e. the end justifies the means. For example, detaining and treating someone in hospital *against their wishes*, to prevent them from committing suicide, would be an example of an action based upon these theories.

Reflective activity

- Which of these two theories do you agree with most closely? Why?
- Which best reflects your organisation and the views of your colleagues?

There are also important principles that underpin good ethical practice in nursing, and healthcare more widely, although there are some different approaches taken, as Box 5.2 indicates.

Box 5.2 Principles of healthcare

Ethical or moral principles of healthcare

There is general agreement that the following four principles underpin ethical behaviour in healthcare:

1. *Non-maleficence* – Do no harm, e.g. do not injure a service user when providing care and treatment.
2. *Beneficence* – Do good, e.g. provide care and treatment that will improve a service user's illness or condition.
3. *Autonomy* – Respect for self-determination, e.g. always respect a service user's wishes and decisions about their treatment (though the MHA or MCA may affect this).
4. *Justice* – Treat people fairly, e.g. do not deny one service user care or treatment that is provided to another service user if they have the same illness or condition.

Virtues

Somewhat by contrast, a virtues approach emphasises the moral character of the individual and the virtues they need, depending upon their role or the situation. These can complement the principles above and can include:

- *Compassion* – the ability to empathise, understand and not judge.
- *Humility* – remembering that we don't have all the answers.
- *Fidelity* – a commitment to help others even if that help is rejected.
- *Justice and courage* – treating people fairly may also require speaking out or protecting them, even at possible cost to oneself.

Ethics of care

There have been some criticisms made of the approaches described above as they are seen not to take into account the involvement and relationships

(continued)

between a practitioner and a service user, or oppressive/discriminatory practice that affects whole cultures or groups (which some argue include people with mental health problems, conditions, or learning disabilities). This ethical approach emphasises the importance of understanding these processes and dynamics to help guide practice, rather than using principles or individuals characteristics alone (see the example of Lisa for an application of virtues and 'ethics of care').

Further reading

Hope, T. (2004) *Medical Ethics: A Very Short Introduction.* Oxford: Oxford University Press.

Scenario: Lisa

Lisa is 21 years old. Her parents are of Jamaican origin but she has no contact with them. She lives in a probation hostel because she has been convicted of shoplifting. She is going out with a man living in the hostel but there is a suspicion that he may hit her although Lisa denies this. She does not work and supplements her benefits by sex working. She uses street drugs. Recently she has been behaving strangely, not caring for herself, acting in a very disinhibited way, and repeating the phrase that 'Is this what grandmother wanted?'. She has been seen stubbing cigarettes out on her arm. Hostel staff want her to move to another hostel. She has agreed to go to A&E where she is seen by a psychiatric nurse but she is very guarded and quite hostile.

If you were that nurse, how can you demonstrate in your practice the following characteristics?:

- *Compassion* – Try and show empathy and understanding and do not judge her because of her lifestyle.
- *Humility* – It will take time to build trust so be careful not to rush in with suggestions about what Lisa needs.
- *Fidelity* – Persevere despite the hostility because all the evidence suggests that Lisa has very significant needs.
- *Justice and honour* – You may have to advocate on behalf of Lisa to the hostel staff to enable her to stay if that is what is best for her even if it makes you unpopular with the hostel staff.
- *Ethics of care* – There is good evidence to show that some people from Black, Asian and minority ethnic communities have experienced racism and discrimination when using mental health services. Sex workers, people with substance misuse problems and offenders have often been excluded from mental health services because they are perceived to be 'difficult' or 'undeserving'. Be aware that Lisa may have experienced these dynamics in the past and recognise the importance of ensuring they do not arise in relationship with services in the future.

Ethics, principles and values in practice

General principles and ethical approaches are not the only dimensions to ethics and values which it is important to be aware of and take into consideration as a nurse. Look at Table 5.1. This outlines several sources of what we usually understand 'values' to mean, that apply to mental health nursing. In some cases these are expressed as values, e.g. the values of an organisation. In other cases, the values are expressed through principles, e.g. in legislation.

Reflective activity

Can you add some examples of what others involved in a person's care may value, e.g. families, other professionals and staff?

Most of the principles and values listed in Table 5.1 should be familiar to you. There appear to be a number of shared values, such as 'respect' and 'dignity'. But there may also be differences in how some of the principles and values are defined. For example, 'recovery' could be defined as 'getting better' or 'cured' but it also may mean 'having more control' or better 'managing' a problem. In practical terms, the aim of 'recovery' may be symbolised for a healthcare professional by a service user leaving hospital. For the service user, the aim may be better symbolised by returning to work, or being able to walk the dog again.

Reflective activity

Think about the principles in Table 5.1 and the two ethical theories described on pp. 92–3.

- Can you personally identify with some of these principles and one of the ethical theories?
- Have an informal discussion with colleagues to find out which principles and ethical theories they believe to be important.
- What possible conflicts exist between the different principles and theories?
- How might these be resolved?

Ethics, principles and values: challenges

Ensuring your work as a mental health nurse is ethical, and based upon sound principles and values, will often be difficult for a number of reasons:

- Principles, ethics and values do not necessarily complement each other, and sometimes they are in direct contradiction. For example, respect for a person's autonomy cannot be at the expense of allowing them to do harm to others.

Table 5.1 Working with value diversity: some sources of principles and values

Principles in the Mental Health Act (MHA) and Mental Capacity Act (MCA)	Relevant principles in the Human Rights Act (HRA) and Equality Act (EA)	Principles in the Nursing and Midwifery Code of Conduct	Healthcare ethics	Organisational policies and good practice	Examples of what service users may value (you may know more)
The MHA Purpose Least restriction Respect Participation Effectiveness, efficiency and equity **The MCA** Assumption of capacity Practical help to make decisions Unwise decisions Best interests Less restrictive	**The HRA** Right to life Prohibition of degrading treatment Right to liberty Right to respect for private and family life **The EA** Prohibition against direct or indirect discrimination on the basis of age, disability, gender reassignment, race, religion or belief, sex, sexual orientation	Treat people as individuals Respect confidentiality Collaborate Ensure consent Maintain professional boundaries Share information Work as part of a team Manage risk Use the best evidence Deal with problems Act with integrity and impartiality	Autonomy Beneficence Non-maleficence Justice Virtues Ethics of care	Respect Dignity Choice and control Empowerment 'Recovery' approach Person-centred Therapeutic benefit Evidence-based Risk averse/positive risk-taking Principles of end-of-life care Principles of clinical governance	Respect Dignity Optimism Ability to manage power imbalances Flexibility Openness Empathy and care Trust Support Empowerment Ability to work across boundaries Ability to 'let go' of the user A nurse's values and attitudes are more than their skills Nurses understand social and other non-medical factors

- Principles and values seem to be everywhere and will certainly be held by others, including other professionals and staff, managers, service users, their families and friends, communities, organisations, and contained in the law itself. In addition to the professional values we have discussed, people's gender, race, age, ethnicity, sexual orientation, disability, cultural background, religious/spiritual belief, political convictions, or chosen lifestyle may all influence or be the source of an individual's values.
- There are significant examples of psychiatry (including mental health nursing) being used politically in abusive ways, particularly under some oppressive governments (e.g. Nazi Germany). Part of the reason for the closure of the large asylums in the UK was because of evidence of institutional neglect and abuse (e.g. Ely Hospital, Cardiff). People with mental health problems, conditions or disabilities often experience stigma and discrimination. The over-medicalisation of mental distress perceived by many people, and the low quality of care in some hospitals and care homes (as well as the community) remain of real concern. Many people with mental health problems and people with learning disabilities are very mistrustful of mental health services – even when your practice is embedded in sound values and ethics, you may encounter mistrust or hostility.
- Psychiatry and the use of mental health law may sometimes be experienced, particularly by service users and families, as an exercise in power without much evidence of principles or ethics. There may be justifiable reasons for this such as the urgency of the situation. However, the exercise of power can be an expression of conflicting values. It may be considered necessary for the service user's benefit to medicate or seclude someone, prevent them from leaving hospital or a care home, persuade them to participate in a therapeutic activity, etc. but the service user involved may fundamentally disagree and experience these interventions very negatively. Exercising a 'duty of care' may be experienced as being overly protective or paternalistic. Both perspectives may have legitimacy and the law may be correctly applied, yet still be experienced by a service user as disrespectful, undignified, stigmatising, discriminatory or oppressive.
- Statements of values (e.g. by organisations) and codes of ethics do not always provide very helpful guides for dealing with conflicting values in complex situations, especially where a law is involved.

Ethics, principles and values: in practice

Faced with these complex challenges, how does a mental health nurse working in a busy environment decide the best course of action? Lakeman examines these issues more thoroughly and in his discussion of ethical decision-making presents 12 key questions that may need to be considered when assessing situations involving these dilemmas (see Box 5.3). Some of the questions will be easier to answer than others. Those questions in italics are likely to be the more challenging ones, particularly when the MHA or the MCA is being used. That is because they are explicitly about values, or involve other people who may have different values to yours (as opposed to more factual aspects of the decision contained in the other questions).

Box 5.3 Lakeman's 12 questions

1. What is the situation?
2. *Who has an interest in the outcome of the decision and what are their views on the right courses of action?*
3. *What are the choices you have?*
4. *What may be the possible consequences of each choice?*
5. What resources are required for each course of action?
6. *How might each choice affect relationships with others?*
7. *What principles or values stand to be compromised by each choice?*
8. *What principle or value should take precedence in this situation?*
9. What are the rights of the parties involved?
10. What duties arise from these rights?
11. What are the legal requirements in the situation?
12. *Who ought to be involved in decision-making?*

(Barker 2009, Chapter 69, 'Ethics and nursing')

Values-based practice

A different type of approach to these challenges involves placing the emphasis back on values, but focusing on 'good process' rather than establishing 'the right values' (see Woodbridge and Fulford 2004). A very simple exercise to begin to illustrate this is given in the Reflective activity below.

Reflective activity

1. Make a list of any words or short phrases you associate with the word 'values'. Ask some colleagues to do the same. Don't think about it too hard or worry about what the 'right' answers might be.
2. Compare your lists. Are there differences?
3. Try combining the lists. How easy is it to do? Are there any that are rejected?

The exercise may well have resulted in different lists but you could probably agree with colleagues that nearly everything could go into a combined list. This indicates an important element that underpins a values-based approach;

- In values-based practice, values are best understood as 'words which guide actions or decisions'.
- Values can therefore seem quite complex because:
  - there are lots of them;
  - some may vary with time and place but others are unchangeable;

  - they may vary from person to person.
- Despite their complexity, values are not chaotic and, a bit like an extended family, are made up of many members, are *coherent* (although that doesn't mean there aren't differences!).

This may make people who want things to be nice and clear feel uncomfortable. We all like clarity when we are doing things. But there is evidence to show that people working in mental health are a lot less consistent and clear about their values than we might expect.

An important piece of research by Colombo et al. (2003) showed that different groups of professionals, service users and carers presented with the same case study often had very different explanations for mental distress. Another piece of research showed that staff may provide different care or treatment to others compared to what they would like to receive if they were a service user (Mental Health Foundation 2009).

These examples of differences in values are not necessarily a cause for worry or concern. On the contrary, it is potentially very positive. It shows that in mental health work, there is a diversity of values and if this diversity is reflected in staff teams it can be used as a positive asset and resource for good practice and working with service users. This is because it broadens understanding and creates opportunities to engage with service users (and carers), whose values and beliefs may be shared with some staff but not others. Certainly values must not be ignored because they matter to people (whether they are professionals or service users).

What the research also indicates is that people, including professionals, may shift in their views of mental distress depending upon the context and the presenting problem. It indicates that there will not always be agreement about the reasons why someone has become unwell or what is the best course of action to take. A doctor may well use medical terminology in a general discussion about psychosis, for example, but in an assessment of someone with psychotic symptoms may identify more pressing social issues to be dealt with first, see the example of Boban.

Scenario: Boban: a medical or social problem?

Boban is a 25-year-old man from Eastern Europe. He has been sleeping rough on the streets for several weeks. His physical health is poor and he has been observed talking to himself and waving his arms around for no apparent reason. The police have contacted the local mental health service requesting that he be taken to hospital. When he is assessed, it is clear that he has psychotic symptoms but refuses the offer of treatment or to go to hospital. He says he would be willing to go into a hostel. Despite concerns about his mental health, it is agreed that his need for accommodation should be addressed first. A place is found for Boban in a hostel and it is agreed that mental health and hostel staff will monitor him closely to see if his mental state changes. It is thought that he may be more willing to consider treatment once he has accommodation but if he doesn't, and his mental state deteriorates, then consideration will be given to formally assessing him under the Mental Health Act.

It is vital that mental health nurses (and other staff) are aware of diversity of values and possible shifts taking place in their own practice and the practice of others according to circumstance. Clear honest communication, listening to, and respecting other points of view, and safe, open discussion are essential. Being open to different explanations and courses of action when the causes of someone's distress are unclear is crucial. Changing one's mind as more information becomes available is fine – it's about fitting an appropriate explanation (or explanations) to the service user, not 'fitting' the service user to a fixed explanation just to prove the legitimacy of that explanation. This is particularly important where the law is being used to legitimate care or treatment. But the benefits of working in this way are likely to be significant, including improved working relationships with colleagues and more positive relationships with service users and carers. Box 5.4 reminds us that this is just as important when working with people with dementia or learning disabilities, as it is with people with mental health problems.

Box 5.4 Severe dementia and severe learning disabilities: an absence of values?

In the past, people with severe dementia or severe learning disabilities have often been regarded as having lost or lacking in any significant, communicable views of the world they live in and the care they receive. Because of this it has been assumed that people do not have wishes and feelings or beliefs and values, nor do they often have value – in other words, they have been grossly infantilised or regarded as sub-human. This has led to some appalling abuse and neglect, including the mass killing of people with learning disabilities in Nazi Germany and enforced sterilisation programmes in Sweden from the 1930s until the 1950s.

Fortunately these views are much less common, and the practices they gave rise to are largely a thing of the past, though it remains important to be vigilant as discriminatory and derogatory opinions still exist in wider society. There is an increasing body of evidence to demonstrate that people with severe dementia or learning disabilities are able to express wishes and feelings, beliefs and values, often in the form of likes and dislikes. In the 1990s, the work of Tom Kitwood in the field of dementia, in developing and promoting the concept of *personhood* and *person-centred care*, and Eric Emerson in promoting *person-centred planning* for people with learning disabilities have been very influential in achieving this shift (Kitwood 1997; Emerson et al. 2005). Similarly, work on *quality of life* has indicated that people with severe dementia or severe learning disabilities are also able to express views about what is important to them (e.g. Alzheimer's Society 2010). The role of close family and friends, as well as people such as advocates, has also been very important in communicating to professionals and other staff what a person's likes and dislikes are when they are unable to do this for themselves.

From the previous discussion we can identify other important elements to values-based practice:

- Values are subjective but as we are about to see, so is much of psychiatry. It is therefore essential to understand the points of views and perspectives of all those directly involved in any given decision or course of action - as well as using evidence from observation and research.
- Good nursing practice (and decision-making in mental health in general) are not about saying whose values are 'right' because this is likely to exclude the values of others as being 'wrong'. Of course, there are certain limits to this and the next section addresses this. Nevertheless it needs to incorporate working with a wide diversity of values, even if that may feel a bit uncomfortable at times. The key is ensuring 'good process' when confronted by a diversity of values.

Limits to values-based practice?

Values-based practice does not mean that 'anything goes'. Where someone's values cause them to act in ways that clearly infringe on the rights or lives of others, then values-based practice must occur within the wider legal framework. Clear examples of this arise where people's actions contravene the principles in the MCA or MHA, infringe the articles in the Human Rights Act, are discriminatory under the Equality Act, or are contrary to other civil or criminal law. Consider the scenario of Mrs Smith.

Scenario: Mrs Smith

Mrs Smith is a white woman, aged 89 years, who has lived all her life in the Essex countryside. She has been diagnosed with dementia and now lives in a care home. She frequently shouts racist abuse at other residents and staff who are Black or Asian but does not like to be left on her own in her room. She claims they steal her possessions though nothing has ever gone missing from her room or her person. Her notes indicate that she did have a purse snatched by an Asian youth shortly before she moved into the home. Mrs Smith has recently developed leg ulcers but refuses to see the GP who visits the home and is Chinese. Recently she became very confused, believing herself to have died and gone to heaven, and hit an Asian resident.

- Is she infringing the rights of other residents or is her verbal abuse of other residents and staff just an unpleasant aspect of her dementia that has to be tolerated?
- How far should her own experiences of race and ethnicity be explored and understood?
- Is her refusal to see the doctor due to a lack of capacity or simply an unwise decision based upon her own prejudice?

(continued)

- What action do you think should be taken as a result of the most recent incident? Which laws might help in this situation and how?

Now imagine there is no element of racism in this scenario at all but Mrs Smith still shouts abuse, believing other residents and staff to be certain members of her family. Her nephew stole her purse. She refuses to see the GP because she thinks he's her father.

Would your responses be different?

The example of Mrs Smith is a complex, but not uncommon one. Values-based practice should still take place using 'good process', but this needs to occur in the context of using both the principles of good nursing care as well as possibly elements of the law, to reduce her distress and the distress of other residents (and potentially staff too).

Values-based practice and the law

'Values-based practice' is therefore based upon a different approach to mental health nursing than just trying to care according to the 'right' values. It can work well because it can accommodate a diversity of values and competing values without making people accept that their values are necessarily 'wrong' or 'bad'. However, it may still seem tough to put into practice, particularly when the MHA or the MCA may be needed to provide care or treatment to someone who is resisting or refusing it. It therefore requires a number of key factors to ensure 'good process'. The factors which are of particular relevance when the MHA or the MCA are being used are laid out in Box 5.5 – the first four are fundamental skills for effective nursing. How would you apply each of these seven pointers to the situation involving Mrs Smith described above?

Box 5.5 Seven key pointers in good process in values-based practice

1. *Awareness:* of one's own values and the values of others in a given situation. Careful attention to language is one way of raising awareness of values.
2. *Reasoning:* using a clear reasoning process to explore the values present when making decisions.
3. *Knowledge:* of the values and facts relevant to the specific situation.
4. *Communication:* combined with the previous three skills, clear, open communication with all involved is central to the resolution of conflicts and the decision making process.
5. *Person (service user)-centred:* the first source of information on values in any situation is the perspective of the service user concerned.

(continued)

6 *Multi-disciplinary working:* conflicts of values are resolved not by trying to establish whose perspective is the 'right' one or by applying 'rules' but by working towards a balance of different perspectives (applying points 1 and 4 above is particularly important here).
7 *Values-based practice (VBP) and evidence-based practice (EBP) working together (see below):* VBP does not 'trump' EBP nor need they be in conflict. All decisions should be based on facts *and* values. But difficulties arise if awareness and communication about values do not take place as then they may only appear when there is a problem (like the difficult debates that can occur if someone is rapidly becoming mentally unwell or their behaviour has suddenly become a source of concern and there are differences of opinion about what should be done).

(Adapted from Woodbridge and Fulford 2004)

Values-based practice and evidence-based practice: how can they work together?

Of course, it is very important working in healthcare to ensure that care and treatment provided are based upon sound evidence that it is effective. This is particularly important when care and treatment are being provided to someone who is unable or refuses to give their consent to receiving treatment. Shouldn't care and treatment therefore be provided on the basis of what we *know* to be right, not what we *believe* to be right? Consider the five people described below.

- *Irma* is 77 and has a diagnosis of Alzheimer's disease. Most of the time she is very confused and forgetful, though she is usually cheerful and gives the impression of being quite content. She lives in a residential care home and often tries to go out alone. However, she always gets lost if she goes out on her own and has very little sense of road safety. Irma does not understand the diagnosis that has been given to her and does not like seeing doctors.
- *Mohammed* is 66 and lives alone. His wife died 3 years ago and he was depressed for a very long time. He eventually saw his GP who diagnosed depression and prescribed anti-depressants. Mohammed has also been trying to take regular exercise with a walking group to help himself feel less depressed. Recently he had very bad flu and this made him feel very low again. He has agreed with his GP to go into hospital because of his depression.
- *Carol* is 47 and has been diagnosed with a chronic back condition. This causes her a lot of physical pain and discomfort but she manages to work part-time. She lives alone and manages her condition through a variety of treatments and therapies, including psychological therapy. Carol accepts the diagnosis and finds it helpful in understanding her condition.
- *Derek* is 22 and has a diagnosis of schizophrenia. He has never had any regular employment and lives at home with his parents. When Derek has a psychotic episode he has a deep-seated and complex belief that he has a

duty given to him by God to cure the world of cancer. This belief sometimes causes him to feel suicidal. At other times his beliefs result in him getting angry and shouting threats at people in the street. Derek does not accept the diagnosis that has been given to him.

- *Natalie* is 32 and has a learning disability. She lives in supported accommodation and volunteers regularly at her church. She can make most decisions about her everyday life but understands that she has a disability and that for more complex decisions she sometimes may need help from others.

All five individuals are clearly very different and this will be reflected in the general values they have, or have expressed in the past. But what is different about Irma and Derek, compared to Mohammed, Carol and Natalie, in relation to their diagnoses?

All five have a diagnosed illness, condition or disability. We normally associate illness with objective experiences of pain, discomfort, dysfunction and distress. This is certainly the case for physical illnesses and conditions like Carol's. She has sought treatments for her back condition which she finds helpful. Similarly, Mohammed has experienced distress that he has accepted treatment for and voluntarily gone into hospital. Natalie also understands that she has a disability that she needs some support with at times.

But Irma and Derek, despite being diagnosed with an illness, either do not understand or do not accept that diagnosis. Indeed, an illness such as schizophrenia is only diagnosed by looking at symptoms such as behaviour and cognitive functioning. There is no diagnostic test for schizophrenia that has 100 per cent accuracy or absolute proof of it as an illness. Both Irma and Derek also do not understand or accept that their illnesses may require them to be cared for, or receive treatment. Both of them seem to have their own explanations (though it is harder to know with Irma) for what others see as an illness, and these explanations do not necessarily in their own right cause Irma or Derek pain or distress.

Facts and values in mental illness

The five people above illustrate what Dickenson and Fulford (2001) describe as the 'fact and value' model of mental illness. There are observable 'facts' about all five people's illnesses, conditions or disabilities, in terms of symptoms and behaviours. These facts are the same for Carol and Mohammed, and to a large extent for Natalie, as they would be for a nurse involved in caring for them: at times they are experiencing pain, distress or difficulty and readily accept support and treatment. In other words, there is a *consensus* of values about what is happening and what needs to be done. But for Irma and Derek, that consensus does not exist as their subjective experience of their 'illness' is different to that of an observer and they want to exercise self-determination and independence rather than seek care or treatment.

Irma and Derek also illustrate an important difference between physical illness and mental illness which helps explain the 'fact and value' models of mental illness. There tends to be much greater consensus about the 'facts' of physical illness in terms of identifiable diseases and injuries, and how these are experienced and described by patients in terms of pain, symptoms, etc. Most people would describe the symptoms of a broken leg or fever using similar ('objective') terms. With a mental illness, even with organic diseases like Alzheimer's, there is much less consensus about the 'facts' of the illness because, by definition, the illnesses (and often the care and treatment) are experienced in very personal ('subjective') ways. In other words, their 'values' are automatically brought into play. Although words like 'delusion' or 'confusion' may be used to describe the symptoms of these illnesses, these may not be words the person themselves would use and how one person with a diagnosis of schizophrenia describes their experience of it is likely to be very different to someone else's. Derek and Irma's experiences of their illnesses are unique to them.

Applying values-based practice to the MHA and the MCA

Why is all of this important in relation to the law? Both the MHA and the MCA allow a person to be detained, supervised and treated without their consent because they are unable or unwilling to accept that they are unwell and require care and treatment. These are the most serious situations where there are disagreements about the 'facts' of mental illness and there is a lack of shared values.

If we take Derek as an example, and consider a situation where he has become more suicidal, or more threatening. Because he is deemed to be unwell, but has not actually done anything really bad (or committed a crime), yet disagrees that he is unwell and/or poses a risk (i.e. disagrees about the 'facts' of being unwell), shared values explaining his behaviour or what to do about it do not exist in the same way. However, the 'respect' and 'participation' principles in the MHA code of practice remind staff that the views, wishes and feelings of Derek must be considered (and the views of his family should also be encouraged) when making decisions under the Act. This makes it complex to decide what to do.

Likewise, imagine if Irma gets a nasty but non-serious infection and lacks capacity to make a decision about the treatment she needs. Because she does not like doctors, she refuses to see one. Staff may therefore need to make important decisions about whether she has capacity to refuse to see a doctor and if this is therefore an 'unwise' decision but one that they have to respect. If she lacks capacity, staff have to decide on her behalf about whether it is in her 'best interests' (under the MCA) to see a doctor over and above Irma's dislike of doctors. The best interests 'checklist' in the MCA states that the past and present wishes and feelings, and beliefs and values of Irma must be considered, as well as the views of others such as her family. But the MCA does not tell staff making the decision what is 'right' or 'wrong' in terms of whether or not she *must* see a doctor – it just describes the process for deciding what to do.

Values-based practice provides a process for weighing up the different principles and values underpinning the law, together with all the other values that you need to take into account, to help you come to a balanced decision in any particular situation in practice. Many of these principles and values are identified in Table 5.1 but this is only a guide – you will need to find out about your organisational policies and protocols yourself. More importantly, you need to find out from individual service users that you work with, their families and friends, and your colleagues, what their values are in order to ensure your practice is both ethical and legal – the principles of both Acts explicitly require you to find out the views, wishes and feelings of the person, and in the case of the MCA, their values, wherever possible.

While the principles of the MCA and the MHA must be followed, they may also have to be balanced with each other to support best practice in applying the law, and in keeping with the Codes of Practice. Values-based practice emphasises a balanced decision-making process, which as we shall see, can also be used to help decide which piece of legislation is most appropriate to use in certain situations. Principles and values from other sources, such as service users, will also need to be included in this process.

Reflective activity

1. Look again at the principles that underpin the MHA and the MCA on p. 96.
2. How might these apply to Derek or Irma?
3. Identify the words or phrases that are likely to involve discussions about values, e.g. best interests.
4. What other values may also be important?
5. How could the 'good process' of values-based practice be easily and quickly used to help you decide what to do?

Values-based practice (VBP) therefore is a good way of dealing with situations where there is tension, disagreement or conflict about what to do. But even using all the elements of VBP's 'good process' does not necessarily mean that everyone will be in agreement or happy with the outcome. For example:

- Derek may still disagree with being detained in hospital under the MHA. Derek's family, and other practitioners may also disagree with this.
- Irma's family or some staff may disagree with her unwise decision not to see a doctor if she is found to have mental capacity to decide. Irma may disagree with seeing a doctor under a best interests decision if she is found to lack capacity – and some staff may also disagree that she needs to see a doctor.

As a nurse you may therefore have to acknowledge that you may be doing the 'wrong thing' from the perspective of others, such as where you are acting against the wishes of someone like Derek and involved in their compulsory detention and treatment, but you are doing the 'right thing' in relation to the law. In effect, you are both wrong and right – a key competency for working in situations like these therefore is the ability to hold two contradictory 'truths' in one's mind at the same time (a mark of genius according to the famous writer, F. Scott Fitzgerald!). Furthermore, by being open and honest with Derek, demonstrating respect and empathy for his experience, you may find yourself agreeing that, according to his values and perspective on the world around him, he is 'right'. Your interventions as a nurse may therefore feel 'wrong' for both you and Derek! But rather than become overly defensive of one's actions, VBP emphasises the importance of acknowledging those difficult and uncomfortable situations and bearing in mind that the outcome may in the longer term be positive – perhaps an unusual example of a situation where two wrongs *can* make a right!

Box 5.6 Research indicates . . . that values-based practice can help

'Unwise' decisions

Deciding what an 'unwise' decision is (according to the third principle of the MCA) can be very difficult. VBP helps in understanding the beliefs and values that underlie and explain why an individual is making what you may feel is an unwise decision. Just because there are concerns about someone's 'risky behaviour', or that they are 'non-compliant', or 'lacks insight' about the care and treatment others feel they need, may involve unwise decisions, but is not automatic proof of a lack of capacity.

Assessing capacity

A range of values may affect practice when assessing capacity, for example. Pressures of time and resources may tilt practitioners either in favour of assessing the person as having capacity (and therefore able to give consent to a medical intervention even if they do not properly understand it) or as not having capacity (because it would take too long to explain the intervention and doing it via best interests is easier). VBP can help nurses to be aware of these other values that may place pressure on them, and find ways of addressing them through supervision and team discussions.

Best interests decision-making

VBP can help with best interests decision-making where not only may there be different views about what is the person's best interests but the 'best interests' of others may be raised, such as family carers. The best interests of the individual may be very dependent upon the involvement of others and therefore their views must be heard and taken into consideration. This can particularly be the case where the safety of the individual or family member is an issue.

The MCA does not say what the outcome should be from a best interests decision and sometimes there may be disagreements about this. These can be difficult to deal with and although VBP may help in resolving these disagreements, this will not always be the case. Other processes may have to be used including mediation, complaints procedures, and ultimately asking the Court of Protection to make a ruling. However, it is very important as a nurse involved in these situations to ensure that the *process* of the best interests decision as described in the Code of Practice is correctly followed.

(continued)

Best interests and multi-disciplinary decision-making

The MCA requires there to be a decision-maker for best interests decisions and to be decision-specific but many situations involve consensus or joint decision-making, such as in some multi-disciplinary teams settings and ward rounds, and multiple, complex decisions, such as decisions about hospital discharge. VBP can provide a good process in these situations to ensure that different views are heard, understood, and taken into consideration, as the MCA requires, while at the same time allowing a decision to be made and to be clear who the decision-maker is. Breaking complex decisions down into a series of sub-decisions is important and helpful and may enable the person lacking capacity to participate more.

Advance decisions and statements

Recognise that family members and professionals may not agree with what is in someone's advance decision or statement, but that it should be respected and followed, depending upon its legal status – the process of VBP can help in situations where family members or professionals are in disagreement.

MCA/MHA interface

The vast majority of psychiatric inpatients detained under the MHA lack capacity to consent to their admission and treatment. But people with a diagnosis of a personality disorder or an eating disorder can pose particular challenges as they may present as still having mental capacity to make decisions about care and treatment even if they have been detained under the MHA. Again, the process of VBP may help by enabling a discussion with a service user that acknowledges their views while explaining the reasons for a hospital admission. It also emphasises the importance of supporting service users to create advance decisions and statements when they are well as these may help clarify decisions about care and treatment when they are in crisis.

Conclusion

The MHA and the MCA have clear principles that underpin the ways in which they should be used. In the MHA these principles are contained in the Code of Practice, whereas in the MCA they are written into the law itself. There are also the principles underlying the HRA and Equality Act. It is very helpful when laws are underpinned by principles because these can be incorporated into the balanced decision-making process emphasised by values-based practice, to help guide people such as nurses when they are involved in using the law.

The wishes and feelings, beliefs and values of everyone involved when the MHA or the MCA is being used may vary dramatically. People may say one thing but believe another, there may be different explanations and courses of action suggested by different practitioners, as well as by the service user and by their families and friends. There are also a number of other important factors, principles or requirements of good mental health nursing that need to be taken into account.

Box 5.7 Key challenges in working with the values underlying the MHA and the MCA

- The different sets of values and principles identified in Table 5.1 still apply in most situations even if someone is subject to the MHA or the MCA.
- However, some clearly have the potential to clash (e.g. autonomy vs compulsion under the MHA or the MCA).
- Service users may not experience principles or values such as beneficence, non-maleficence, respect, dignity, person-centred or therapeutic benefit when subject to compulsion under the MHA or the MCA.
- In most situations the principles of the HRA, the EA and the MCA, still apply even if someone is subject to the MHA - and the HRA and the EA apply when the MCA is being used.

Values-based practice (VBP) does not tell you the 'answer' to the dilemmas posed by Table 5.1 and the key challenges in Box 5.7. Nor does it tell you which set of competing factors, principles or requirements are the right ones, though clearly nurses and other staff must always act in accordance with the law. What it does do is encourage honest and open discussion about the various interactions and possible tensions that may exist between them.

In Part II we look at how the MHA and the MCA apply in different situations and settings. We will keep on coming back to values-based practice as a way of helping you think through some of the complexities and dilemmas that these situations and settings pose.

Key points: Summary

- Mental health nursing is different to other types of nursing because mental illnesses, conditions and disabilities have significant differences to physical illnesses – the MHA and the MCA reflect this.
- It is helpful to think of values as 'decision- or action-guiding words'.
- Encountering differences in values, and disagreements over values are inevitable for mental health nurses – especially when you are involved with the MHA or the MCA.
- Values-based practice provides a good way of dealing with those differences and disagreements ('value diversity') – but it doesn't provide the answers!
- Being able to work with 'value diversity' demonstrates your ability to work ethically, as well as where the MHA or the MCA applies, legally.

Part II
Practice

Part II looks at how the MCA and MHA should be applied by mental health nurses in practice, at different stages and in different settings of a service user 'journey'. It starts with service users living in the community, being admitted into hospital, treated and discharged, living in care homes, and the particular ways the law applies for children and young people. The chapters begin with an explanation of how the MCA and MHA apply in theory and then use scenarios to show how they apply in practice. The scenarios involve fictitious service users but are based upon real-life examples from the authors' experience and knowledge.

Reflective questions in each chapter encourage you to think about how the law should be used. Depending upon the setting or stage of the service user journey you are interested in, each chapter provides a description of how the different pieces of legislation apply in practice so you can read the chapters separately, or one by one in succession. Some of the chapters use continuations of scenarios from previous chapters and some use one-off scenarios.

It is important that you refer back to the chapters in Part I and the decision matrix in the Appendix for a more detailed description of the different laws if you are unsure. Items in the text in **bold** refer to key roles, processes, or parts of the different laws - where necessary, use Part I to remind yourself of what they mean.

Use the process described in Chapter 5 on values-based practice to help you think through some of the challenges and dilemmas that applying the law may pose.

6 Working with people living in the community

Learning outcomes

This chapter covers:

- Relevant legal principles and processes when working with individuals living in the community
- Importance of supporting people to make decisions for themselves
- Why and how decisions may need to be made on behalf of people who lack capacity to make a decision for themselves
- Scenarios involving people living in the community who may lack capacity to make decisions for themselves

Introduction

Most people with mental health problems, learning disabilities, dementia, and alcohol and substance misuse problems live in the community. Since the closure of the long-stay hospitals in the 1980s, policy and practice have focused on caring for people in community settings and only using hospital for when people are in crisis. Institutional care (usually care homes) is mainly used for people in the later stages of dementia.

It is essential that you understand how the Mental Capacity Act (MCA) and the Mental Health Act (MHA) apply in community settings. It is also essential that you understand how the MCA and the MHA should 'fit' together when you are working with people living in the community, how other relevant legislation, such as the Human Rights Act (HRA) and the Equality Act (EA), apply, and how values-based practice can help when there are difficulties or disagreements.

This chapter provides a guide to how this legislation should be applied in practice when working with people living in the community. The chapter does *not* cover the specific aspects of the MHA which can be applied to people living in the community (primarily community treatment orders and guardianships) as these are covered in Chapter 9. Nor does it cover how the MCA or the MHA apply when you are considering admitting someone into psychiatric hospital or residential/nursing care as this is covered in Chapter 7 and Chapter 10.

The chapter begins by briefly describing what is meant by 'community' and then outlines some of the key elements of the relevant legislation that apply to people living in the community that you may work with. It then continues with some scenarios looking at how the law affects people living in the community.

Defining 'community'

'Living in the community' can apply to a whole range of activities in a person's life including where they live, what they do during the day (and night), who they see and where they go. As a mental health nurse you may come into contact with people living in the community in a variety of settings. You may meet them in different places:

- where the person lives, e.g. their own home, supported or sheltered accommodation (but see Chapter 10 for people living in care homes), temporary accommodation (e.g. hostels), staying with family or friends, etc.;
- at a community team office;
- in an outpatient's clinic, day hospital or day centre;
- depending upon your role, you may also have contact with people at a place of work, employment or training schemes, education or leisure facilities, in public places such as the street or a park;
- through telephone contact, or through text, email or Skype to maintain contact.

Contact may be part of a routine visit or appointment, an urgent or emergency appointment, or even a random encounter in a public place or while seeing another person.

Reflective activity

- What are the different types of community settings that you are aware of or have experience of working in?
- Are there particular challenges of working in some of those settings?
- How can those challenges be overcome?

Applying legal principles and values-based practice working with people in the community

In community settings all the principles of the Mental Capacity Act (MCA), the Human Rights Act (HRA) and the Equality Act (EA) apply, together with healthcare ethics, principles contained in the NMC code of conduct, and your organisation's policies and procedures. The values and beliefs of the service user, and potentially others involved in their care and support also need to be taken into account. It may feel a bit overwhelming to try and apply all these different principles and values when working as a nurse in the community, especially if they come into conflict. The values-based practice approach described in Chapter 5 can help you in these situations.

Most service users living in their own homes in the community will be able to make most decisions for themselves and as a nurse the **first principle of the MCA** (assumption of capacity) is an important starting point for how you work with people. However, for more complex decisions involving care and treatment issues, or where someone's mental health problem or condition is deteriorating, nurses may need to be more involved in helping someone to make a decision. Providing information in a way that a service can understand, in order to give or refuse consent to care or treatment that you are responsible for providing, is a key task in virtually any encounter with them. The **second principle of the MCA** emphasises the importance of supporting people to make their own decisions. It is also important to remember that people's chosen lifestyles may be quite unusual or eccentric, or very different to what is considered to be 'normal'. The decisions they make about their lives may not be ones that other people would agree with but this is where the **third principle of the MCA** is important (unwise decisions).

However, from time to time, a service user may have difficulty making a decision, despite being given support, or may be making a particularly strange decision about an aspect of their care or treatment that you are providing to them. In these situations it may be necessary to carry out a mental capacity assessment. This must be done in accordance with the MCA. If it shows the person lacks capacity to make the decision, then you can make it in their **best interests**, in accordance with the **fourth and fifth principles of the MCA** and (best interests and **less restrictive principles**) and the best interests process.

If you follow these principles correctly, then you can legally make the decision or provide care or treatment to the person despite them being unable to give their consent, without fear of being held liable. It is essential that you also consider other important factors in mental capacity assessments and best interests decisions (Chapter 2 explains these in more detail):

- Be decision-specific and time-specific.
- Not jumping to conclusions because of age, appearance, condition or behaviour.
- Involve others who know the person, and specialists (where necessary).
- Provide the person with practical and appropriate help to be involved in the decision.
- Base your assessment or decision upon a reasonable belief.
- Make a clear recording of your assessment or decision.

You also need to check if the person has a health and welfare attorney authorised under an **LPA**, a **court-appointed deputy**, an **advance decision to refuse treatment** (ADRT), or is entitled to an **IMCA**. Remember that an attorney, deputy and ADRT can be involved in decisions which may be legally binding on nurses even if a nurse disagrees with them.

Although the MCA is critical in how you practise as a nurse working with people living in the community, you must not lose sight of the other legislation, principles, and ethics of care as outlined in Chapter 2. This may at times be challenging because there may be conflicts in your own mind about how to balance different values, principles or policies, or different and conflicting points of view among those involved. This is where the 'good process' described by values-based practice in Chapter 5 is so important. Unless the situation is an emergency or requires urgent action, then **values-based practice** provides a framework for resolving these issues.

In situations where there is disagreement, a number of approaches can be taken but the three most advisable ones to use are:

- a multi-disciplinary approach and consult with colleagues in your team (although that may be where some of the conflict lies!);
- professional or peer supervision;
- referring the decision to someone with more experience and expertise.

Other approaches could include:

- organising a meeting with all the key players (including the service user and anyone they wish to attend with them unless there are very good reasons for not doing this) to try and reach a consensus
- seeking confidential, external advice, e.g. from the NMC or legal advice
- contacting the **Office of the Public Guardian** in situations involving an LPA or court-appointed deputy
- consulting reliable, good quality guidance and online resources (see Useful Resources on p. 211).

The rest of this chapter presents two scenarios involving using the law with people living in the community, designed to give you some frameworks and ideas for best practice.

Scenario: Atul

Atul is a 22-year-old man who lives in London. His parents are from Pakistan but Atul was born in the UK. He has two brothers and two sisters. He left school at 16 and did a variety of manual jobs but in his late teens started smoking cannabis and taking other illegal drugs.

His GP has referred Atul to a community mental health team where you work. He saw his GP recently, complaining of a constant buzzing in his ears which he thinks may be to do with extra-terrestrials that he said are part of global terrorism. You send Atul an appointment to come and see you and a psychiatrist.

Atul arrives on the day of the appointment and seems worried and agitated. He talks quite openly regarding his beliefs about extra-terrestrials. At the end of the interview the psychiatrist asks Atul to wait and then talks to you in private. The psychiatrist tells you that he believes Atul has a psychotic illness and lacks mental capacity and is therefore going to tell him that he must have an anti-psychotic injection immediately, otherwise Atul will probably need to be admitted to hospital. You don't disagree with the diagnosis but make the following points:

- Although Atul seems to have a psychotic illness, this does not mean that he lacks mental capacity – **mental capacity should be assessed on a decision-specific basis** according to the MCA.

- You therefore suggest starting off by assuming Atul has capacity in accordance with the **first principle of the MCA** and ask for his consent to be given the injection, and to explain why this is being suggested.

The psychiatrist agrees and this is what you do. You explain to Atul that he seems very worried about the extra-terrestrials and that you and the psychiatrist are suggesting that he is given some medication to help him feel less worried. You ask Atul if he agrees to this. Atul asks some questions about the side effects of the medication and gives this some thought. Atul then agrees. You check with Atul that he has understood, retained and weighed up (used) the information involved in the decision (**assessment of capacity**), and it is clear that he has. You are therefore confident that he had the capacity to make this decision and give his consent so you give him the injection.

Reflective question

What kind of questions might you ask to find out if Atul has capacity to make this decision?

Although Atul has the injection, his subsequent contact with you is very sporadic. Six months later Atul becomes very unwell and has a voluntary admission into psychiatric hospital. Although only a short admission, a year later he is admitted again, presenting as being very psychotic. Following the second admission, Atul moves into supported accommodation where a housing worker visits him and helps him with practical things like his welfare benefits. Atul attends a clinic once a fortnight for a depo injection and over the last year his mental health has been much more stable although it is believed that he continues to take drugs.

It is the day Atul is due to have his injection. Atul arrives but seems quite disoriented. He is vague and ambivalent when you talk to him about the injection, but seems reluctant to have it. He admits that he smoked some cannabis earlier in the day and he also smells of alcohol.

You think that Atul may temporarily lack capacity to give consent to having the injection – this needs assessing according to the MCA and it may be advisable to ask him to wait, see if the effects of the cannabis and alcohol wear off and then reassess his capacity to give consent. After an hour Atul still seems disorientated and is unable to indicate whether he is willing to have the injection or not. His thoughts are wandering and the clinic is about to close. You decide that he lacks capacity to give consent to having the injection **because you have a reasonable belief that he cannot understand, retain and use the information to make the decision**.

Reflective question

What questions might you ask to establish a reasonable belief that Atul lacks capacity to make this decision?

You have to make a **best interests decision**. You ask Atul to wait and you speak to the psychiatrist who is concerned about Atul not having his injection but wants more information and is worried about Atul having the injection on top of alcohol and cannabis. You then phone the housing support worker to ask him how Atul has been – he tells you that Atul has been fine. Taking these views into account, together with his ambivalence and a degree of reluctance as an indication of Atul's wishes and feelings you believe you have considered all the relevant circumstances to make a best interests decision. You decide that it is not in Atul's best interests to have the injection today. As part of this decision you also have to take into account what the consequences are if you do not give Atul the injection.

Reflective questions

- What factors do you have to take into account to do this?
- What might you consider having to do if you decided that he must have the injection today?

You do not give him the injection but explain to Atul that you will visit him at home the next day to see how he is and give him his injection then, if Atul agrees. You are careful to keep a record of what you have done because it is an **action in connection with care and treatment** of Atul and you would therefore be liable for anything that happens (e.g. Atul having a breakdown) if you had not correctly assessed his capacity and acted in his best interests, in accordance with the MCA. You visit Atul the next day and he seems much better and has the capacity to make a decision about his injection – he agrees to have it.

A week later you have organised Atul's CPA meeting. Atul, his mother, his psychiatrist and the housing support worker attend. His mother says that she wants help to move Atul to different accommodation as she is worried that he is taking drugs where he lives at the moment. She says that Atul cannot make decisions for himself because he is unwell and that these should be made on his behalf. The psychiatrist agrees that Atul should move because of the risk that smoking cannabis poses to Atul's mental health. Atul is asked if he wants to move somewhere else. It is not clear that Atul understands or can weigh up all the information involved in making the decision but does repeatedly say he wants to talk to Razia, one of his sisters.

You suggest postponing the decision and having a meeting involving Razia for the following reasons:

- You are unsure if Atul has capacity to make the decision about his accommodation but you think about the first two principles of the MCA – the assumption of capacity and providing help to enable someone to make a decision for themselves. You think that Razia may be able to help Atul make a decision.
- Razia may also be able to provide more information about Atul's capacity to make a decision – while acknowledging the importance of getting everyone's else's view as well.

- If Atul is unable to make the decision, then Razia can help with the best interests decision about where Atul lives.

Everyone agrees except for the mother who is upset that a decision cannot be made then and there and thinks that Razia is a bad influence on Atul and should not therefore be involved. Because Atul has expressed a wish about Razia being present, you explain to Atul's mother that this should be respected. Atul's mother is not happy about this but agrees to come to the meeting providing Razia is not allowed to say too much.

After the meeting the housing support worker tells you that if Atul does not have capacity to make a decision about his accommodation, then this could jeopardise his tenancy agreement which Atul signed on the basis that he had the capacity to make the decision to live there. The worker explains that no -one can make a best interests decision to sign a tenancy agreement on behalf of someone who lacks capacity unless it is an **attorney with an LPA** or **court-appointed deputy** with this authority - Atul has neither of these.

At the meeting involving Razia, Atul seems more relaxed. His mother and the psychiatrist still believe that Atul lacks the capacity to make a decision about where he lives but you mediate the meeting to enable the housing support worker to talk to Atul about his accommodation. Atul listens carefully and Razia sometimes explains what the worker has said in Urdu to Atul. Razia gives you the impression of being helpful and not trying to unduly influence Atul. Atul asks some sensible questions about his tenancy and then states clearly that he does not wish to move. Everyone except his mother agrees that Atul can understand, retain and use the information to make this decision and he therefore has capacity. It is therefore agreed that he will stay where he is although his mother disagrees and the psychiatrist is still worried.

You explain that although they may consider Atul's decision to stay in his tenancy to be an unwise one which they don't agree with, this does not mean he lacks the capacity to make the decision according to the MCA. The psychiatrist still has concerns about Atul's capacity to make a decision about what he does during the day and asks whether **Deprivation of Liberty Safeguards (DoLS)** could be used to place some restrictions on Atul. The housing worker explains that DoLS only apply to people in hospital or living in care homes.

Scenario: David

David is 79 and was diagnosed with Alzheimer's disease a year ago, although it is still at a fairly early stage. He lives alone in his own home in a small village. David was a businessman and retired when he was 60. His wife died three years ago and he has one adult daughter, Mary, who lives 30 miles away with her husband Tom and their family. After he was diagnosed he made a **Lasting Power of Attorney (LPA)** which authorised Mary to make decisions about his property, his money, and health and personal welfare matters, including consent to treatment. Jean, David's neighbour, keeps an eye on him and regularly helps him with meals and looking after his house. David attends a day centre in a nearby town - this has been arranged through his local social services but he pays to attend. He catches a bus to go there. Recently there have been concerns about David's health and welfare – the day centre staff have noticed that he seems more confused and sometimes turns up very late. He also is looking much thinner and in the last few days has said he has had no money to buy food.

You work as part of a community team and David is on your caseload. You visit David at home and although he is quite cheerful and pleased to see you, it is clear that the symptoms of Alzheimer's have got worse. There is no food in the kitchen, he says he has no money and cannot remember when he last saw Mary. You also notice that he has bruising on his face and arms which he is unable to explain. You ask him if it's OK to speak to Mary and he agrees but she does not answer her phone. You then ask him if it's OK to speak to Jean and he agrees.

Reflective question

Getting David's agreement involves an assumption of capacity. What would you do if he refused to give his permission or you were unsure about his capacity to give his permission?

Jean says that Mary told her that she had registered the LPA several weeks ago and was now responsible for David's money, and last visited a week ago. She also has concerns about David but has been unable to contact Mary. You have concerns about the possibility of financial abuse by Mary, and even the possibility of physical abuse by someone on David. This is extremely serious as an adult safeguarding issue, and if abuse is occurring, the **Office of the Public Guardian** (OPG – where the LPA is registered), as well as local social services need to be contacted. If there is evidence of deliberate ill-treatment or wilful (intentional) neglect, the person responsible could be prosecuted under the **criminal offence** in the MCA.

Reflective questions

- Do you know what the NMC's Code of Conduct says about adult abuse and safeguarding?
- What is your organisation's policy on it?

You talk to David and explain that you are worried about him and that you want to contact local social services to get him more help. David gets quite upset and says he doesn't want you to do this. You assume that David has capacity to refuse permission and you try to explain as simply as possible why you need to contact social services, in keeping with the first two principles of the MCA. However, you also use this conversation to assess his capacity and quickly come to the conclusion that he may not have capacity to give his consent and therefore you may say his refusal is not simply an unwise decision **(third principle**

of the MCA). You invite Jean to come in (with David's permission) and discuss it more. Even with Jean helping, it is clear that David is unable to understand and weigh up the information to make the decision, so he therefore lacks the capacity to give his permission. You therefore have to make a best interests decision regarding contacting local social services.

Reflective question

What would you do if you assessed David as having capacity?

Although you are mindful of the Human Rights Act (especially Article 8 – the right to privacy and family life) and David's expressed wishes and feelings, you discuss this with Jean and both agree that it is in David's best interests that you contact social services.

Reflective question

What other Articles in the Human Rights Act do you need to be especially mindful of?

You are careful to keep a record of what you have done because it is an **action in connection with care and treatment** of David. You would be liable for anything that happens (e.g. David making a complaint that you had broken confidentiality and infringed his right to privacy) if you had not correctly assessed his capacity and acted in his best interests, in accordance with the MCA.

Reflective question

What would you need to record and where?

You contact David's care manager in social services and they agree to arrange a meeting and speak to the adult safeguarding team. At this stage you agree not to contact the OPG. The care manager also manages to briefly speak to Mary over the phone who sounds quite distressed but agrees to come to the meeting. You discuss with the care manager about making a referral to the local **Independent Mental Capacity Advocate (IMCA)** because although it is not a situation where an IMCA *must* be involved, an IMCA *can* be involved in adult safeguarding situations with a person who lacks capacity, even if the person has family or friends who can be consulted (because as in this situation, it may be that they are responsible for the abuse). However, because of the urgency of the case and Jean's involvement (who is also coming to the meeting, as well as someone from the day centre), you agree not to refer at this stage.

Reflective question

In what situations must an IMCA be involved?

At the meeting (which David attends) the safeguarding issue is not raised directly but you speak of your concerns about David. Mary is very upset and apologetic because she explains that her husband had been involved in a serious car accident a few days ago. She says that she had spoken to David who had said that he was managing OK so she had postponed her visit but knew about her responsibilities as an attorney. She showed David's recent bank statements that indicated withdrawals corresponding with the amount of money David had been getting. Jean also says that since your visit David had told her that he had fallen over and while she was there, he had accidentally burnt himself on the kettle. It is agreed that both David and Mary need much better arrangements if David is to continue living safely at home, so a further care assessment will take place. The care manager asks David if he agrees to this but the care manager decides that David lacks the capacity to give his consent because of his age and behaviour. The care manager therefore asks Mary, as his attorney, to give consent on David's behalf, which she does.

Reflective questions

- Is this a correct way of assessing capacity?
- What would you do if you disagreed with an attorney's (or colleague's) assessment of mental capacity?
- How could a situation be resolved where an attorney refuses consent for the person to have care or treatment provided because the attorney believed it was not in the person's best interests?

After the meeting, you and the care manager agree that the safeguarding concerns are unfounded.

At the care assessment it is decided that David's care package should be increased. It is agreed that a paid carer from a care agency will visit David on a daily basis to help him prepare a hot meal, or make sure he gets to the day centre on the days he attends, and to keep an eye on him. You agree to visit more regularly to monitor the effect of his Alzheimer's. Mary and Jean agree to visit him at weekends.

For several months this care package works well although to start off with Mary and David tell you that he doesn't like the paid carer because she never asks him to decide what he wants to eat. You mention this to the care manager and point out that the MCA emphasises that mental capacity is **decision-specific** – even if he lacks capacity to make complex decisions, it should still be assumed that he can make decisions like this. The paid carer is told this and agrees always to ask David to make the decision about which meals he has.

Key points: Summary

- The MCA applies to everyone living in the community aged 16 and over.
- Most people living in the community will have mental capacity to make decisions for themselves about their lives and the care and treatment they receive. Even if they make unwise decisions, nurses should not assume this means the person lacks capacity.
- Sometimes people may have difficulties making decisions and it is important for nurses to support people to make decisions by providing them with information about the decision that they can understand and by meeting any particular communication needs that they have.
- If a person lacks capacity to make a decision about their care and treatment, then the decision can be made on their behalf in their best interests. The MCA describes a process for deciding what is in a person's best interests and this includes legal safeguards. If this involves the provision of care or treatment, then nurses should be involved in the best interests decision.
- Some people may have expressed their wishes in advance or have appointed someone to make decisions on their behalf if they lack capacity. The MCA provides different way of doing this including advance decisions to refuse treatment and lasting powers of attorney.

7 Admitting people into hospital

Learning outcomes

This chapter covers:

- Different routes by which a person might be admitted to hospital
- The role of the MHA or the MCA in admitting a person and when DoLS is relevant
- The processes involved in admission and the statutory roles of different people

Introduction

In this chapter we will consider the point at which people are admitted to hospital and how the law applies at this point, and who it applies to. The different groups of people include the 250,000 patients being admitted into psychiatric care in hospitals during any one year in UK, people who live in some form of residential care but need to be admitted to hospital, and people who lack capacity being admitted to general hospitals. For some people it will be their first admission; others will be already known to in-patient psychiatric services.

Hospital or care home?

Hospitals and care homes typically cater for different populations of people or for those with different mental health problems. Different hospital settings cater for people who are acutely ill and/or who need to be assessed/treated in a safe environment; in a specialist mental health unit, in a general hospital, in a psychiatric hospital. The 'special hospitals' provide for patients who, in most cases, have been in contact with the criminal justice system but who have been sent to a hospital for assessment or treatment on account of their mental disorder. Depending on the level of security attached to the hospitals, they will be called variously 'high', 'medium' or 'low' secure units.

A care home or nursing home is more likely to care for people who stay longer term, and have chronic mental health conditions or difficulties such as dementia, learning difficulties or brain damage. However, their patients may need to be admitted to hospital for assessment or treatment if their health condition warrants it.

Of course, individuals come with various personal and medical conditions and differing needs, which are themselves changing. Their mental capacity may fluctuate. People may move from one type of institutional care to another or from one level of care to another. So they may be subject to the MCA at one time, DoLS or the MHA at another. Hospital resources and practices differ in different parts of the country. All of these factors will influence the patients you will work with and which legislation applies to their admission for care and treatment.

Hospitals that take detained patients must be registered for that purpose and are regulated and monitored by specific powers given to the Care Quality Commission (England) and the Healthcare Inspectorate (Wales). The CQC also monitors care homes registered under the Care Standards Act 2010.

Reflective activity

Think of the in-patient settings where you have worked so far or are likely to work where there may be patients who will be under the MHA or the MCA or under DoLS. Think how their situation may alter over time.

The named nurse

All service users in hospital must have a **named nurse**, according to the Patients' Charter (DOH 1991), who will be allocated to each individual, within the first 24 hours of their admission. Their role is to coordinate the nursing care, working together with the multi-disciplinary team. It gives the nurse the opportunity to maximise the therapeutic value of the nurse-patient relationship and to foster trust and collaborative working. It may involve a relationship with the patient across several episodes in hospital.

The named nurse should do the following:

- maintain a high level of communication and cooperation between everyone involved in the person's care and treatment (including the community care coordinator if there is one);
- attend multi-disciplinary CPA review meetings, prepare reports and attend Tribunals and Hospital Managers' Hearings;
- take responsibility for all documentation about the implementation of a comprehensive clinical assessment and care plan. This includes ensuring there is a written record of the care programme, of contacts with the service user and carers' views about the content of care programme.
- monitor the progress of the individual, and pass on issues of concern to those involved in their care.

The named nurse should positively address issues raised by the service user and make these known to those involved in their care, especially if the individual feels unable to do this (see e.g. North East London NHS Trust 2010).

Box 7.1 Duties of the named nurse

Matters that may involve the named nurse at the time when a person is admitted under the MHA include:

- holding powers;
- assisting with knowledge of the nearest relative;
- providing information about legal rights;
- helping obtain an advocate;
- compiling the documentation required by law.

Being admitted to hospital

Pathways to hospital

You may work in a hospital psychiatric unit or possibly A&E, and need to decide on whether a hospital admission is required. You may be a community mental health nurse working in a community-based team and needing to find a place in an in-patient unit. You may have in your care an informal patient who needs to be detained.

In all these instances you will be responsible for caring for service users who have become acutely ill – in distress, fearful, confused, suicidal or violent. Or you may need to admit an elderly person to a nursing home because they are no longer able to cope at home. Relatives may be supportive or resistant to the change.

Knowledge of the legislation will assist you to work confidently, apply the law correctly, and communicate effectively with these service users and their carers or family members. You will need to consult them, inform them of what is happening and why, and to explain what their rights are.

Informal patients

People may enter hospital for treatment for mental illness in the same way as they might for their physical illness. They are free to leave when they choose and they may refuse to accept treatment they do not want. If they lack capacity to consent to treatment, they can be treated in their best interests. However, if they then begin to object to treatment, they may discharge themselves or the MHA, the MCA or the DoLS may be needed depending on whether the treatment is for mental or physical disorder. You may even need to exercise the nurses' holding power.

Capacity

The first step will be to assess the person for their **capacity** and for their mental state. The two-stage capacity test is described in Chapter 1. You must remember that the person may lack capacity to decide about whether to be in hospital, where to live, or what treatment they need. However, they may have capacity to decide which family members they want to see or, for example, who they want to take care of their pets. In all cases you must support them to make their own decisions. You should delay the decision wherever possible so the person can make it for themselves (e.g. waiting for someone to sober up) and you should consult with others who know the person.

If, however, the person does lack capacity to consent to admission, the NHS may need to appoint an IMCA to represent them.

Box 7.2 IMCAs and admission to hospital under s.38 MCA

If an NHS body proposes to make arrangements for accommodation in a hospital or care home or for a change to another hospital or care home for a person who lacks capacity to agree to the arrangements, and there is nobody else (other than those providing care or treatment in a professional or paid role with whom it would be appropriate to consult about the person's best interests), an **IMCA** must be appointed to represent them.

What is in the service user's best interests?

Let us return to the stories of Atul and David from Chapter 6 and introduce Sylvia and Alice in order to demonstrate how capacity and **best interests** might work in different circumstances.

Scenario: Atul (see p. 116)

A year after the meeting about Atul's accommodation Atul fails to attend for his fortnightly anti-psychotic injection. You phone the housing worker who says she is worried. She believes he has been smoking cannabis and he is eating little. He no longer attends the drop-in facility at the community centre and seems to stay in his room all day. He is scared of the extra-terrestrials whom he says hang around outside the room. You speak on the phone to him and arrange to visit the next day. He allows you to enter his room. He is slumped in his chair, muttering to himself. You tell him you would like to give him an injection and he pushes you away. You decide he lacks capacity to make the decision to have the injection. You go back to the community team and there is a discussion with other members. The **AMHP** then contacts his sister, Aisha, to see if she can persuade him to have the injection or if not, to go to hospital, and she comes to the house – but he still resists an injection. Further discussion with his psychiatrist follows. She is clear that there is no alternative way to administer his medication and that it is necessary to take him to hospital. Is it in his best interests to go to hospital? You both believe Atul is ill, vulnerable and at risk if he stays in the community, so you ask him what he would like. He does not reply. You tell him that he will be safer in hospital and that you and the doctor will protect him against what he fears will happen. He does not dissent to this but still seems not to understand. You then talk to the doctor about the need for a bed. It is decided that he must go in an ambulance because he is too agitated to be conveyed in a car. When the ambulance arrives, he cannot be persuaded to leave the house. While it would be permissible under the MCA to use mild **restraint** by holding him firmly by the arm, in order to convey him to the ambulance, this would not be effective. To use greater restraint on a person who is so distressed and afraid would not be in his best interests. So the nurse and team decide it would be better to return tomorrow and you tell him that and hope that he may feel better about it the following day. (Had it been an emergency to admit him because of the seriousness of his illness, the police would have been called to accompany him to hospital.)

Scenario: David (see p.119)

David's health declines and his Alzheimer's gets worse. In his confused state he is forgetting to eat and he neglects his hygiene. He is emaciated and withdrawn. He needs to be admitted to the hospital for an **assessment, care and treatment**. Enquiries are made about a bed in the local hospital where there is a joint elderly and psychiatric assessment ward. Mary and you visit David and tell him of the proposal. Mary assures him that she will visit every day and that she will accompany him to the hospital. While it is not clear that he has fully grasped the need for his admission, David understands that he is going into a hospital for the doctors to look after him and to help him feel better. He is assessed as having capacity to make the decision about admission to hospital.

Scenario: Sylvia

Sylvia lives in supported accommodation. She has a learning disability. She is admitted to A&E after she is discovered by a support worker to have cut both her arms deeply. This is the second time in 6 months that she has been admitted for this reason. After her wounds are dressed, you comfort her and listen to her story about the people she does not like where she lives. Later you assist a doctor in doing a full psychosocial assessment. The assessment covers her **capacity to consent to treatment**, her mental state, the nature and degree of risk, and a needs assessment. Having decided that she lacks capacity, you assess that it is in her best interests to be in a psychiatric unit in hospital, to keep safe and to recuperate psychologically and physically from a serious wound. After some discussion she reluctantly agrees to stay in the hospital so she is admitted as an informal patient. The care plan highlights the need to investigate further the living situation and to involve her key worker in that.

Scenario: Alice

Alice, aged 86, is in a care home and suffers from depression. Her recurrent urinary tract infection has returned and she is having difficulty breathing. She has a high temperature and has not responded to antibiotics. Her GP visits and considers that she needs to be admitted to hospital for assessment and treatment. She is feverish and unable to take part in any discussions about the plan so she lacks capacity to make that decision. Both the GP and the senior nurse do not believe that they should delay in the hope that her capacity might return – her condition is more likely to worsen. The reasons for deciding she lacks capacity and the reasons for the best interests decision to admit her are recorded in her medical notes and she is conveyed to the general hospital under the MCA.

Reflection on the scenarios

Atul, Sylvia and Alice were found to have lost capacity to make a decision about admission to hospital and the decision to admit them was taken in their **best interests** under the MCA.

In none of these scenarios would it be necessary to use the DoLS because the people did not need to be deprived of liberty. If Atul or Sylvia objected to treatment for their mental disorder, whether or not they were found to have capacity at the time, the use of the MHA would be considered.

In the case of Alice, the situation is more complex. Although she has been diagnosed with depression, her hospital admission is for her physical condition. If she resisted being taken to hospital, the MCA gives the authority to restrain her using force proportionate to any harm to herself. If that was insufficient force because she struggled and was upset by the restraint, the better course would be to let her remain and contact family or others to help to calm her and persuade her to leave the care home. If, however, this failed, there should be a full discussion with the clinical team before restraint is used. If it became clear that she would need to be restrained in conveying her to hospital, the **DoLS Code of Practice** recommends an application to the **Court of Protection** would ensure that the conveyance was lawful (DoLS Code of Practice 2.15).

Detention: Admission under the MHA

Values-based practice

Values-based practice goes to the heart of what is so difficult about compulsion:

> In most situations throughout health and social care, while those involved may have some differences of values (for example, about what is the best treatment to use from different points of view), usually they should be working together to the same ends. But with compulsory treatment there is a direct clash of values. In short, the person concerned wants one thing (not to be treated) while everybody else wants the opposite (that s/he gets treatment).
>
> (DH Guidance)

The values in conflict when it comes to detaining somebody are, on the one hand:

- respect for the person's human rights to freedom and autonomy and the need to place their wishes and values at the heart of their treatment;
- non-discrimination between mental and physical illness;

and on the other hand:

- the rights of people to be kept safe and to be treated when their judgement is impaired by their illness;
- the rights of others to be safe from violence.

There is still a stigma attached to being detained. The service user stands to lose a lot as a result – home, jobs and family relationships can be jeopardised. While many people are grateful in retrospect for their having been kept safe at a time when they did not know how unwell they were and what was best for them, others look back on it as having done them harm. Indeed, a recent English study found that only 40 per cent of detained patients who took part in the study considered, 12 months after leaving hospital, that their detention had been justified (Priebe 2009). Some service users state that the trauma of being detained affected them for years and made them fearful of doctors and hospitals.

The MHA and the MCA principles are the most important guides for balancing these competing values. While the new **MHA Code of Practice** no longer uses the phrase that compulsion should be the last resort, the principle in favour of the **least restrictive option** makes a similar point. Take Atul, for example:

- By talking to Atul in a way that he could understand and listening to his fears about the extra-terrestrials, he was comforted and his fears about leaving his room were overcome. He trusted the doctor and AMHP to keep him safe as long as they were with him and to look after him, so he was able to receive care and treatment without being detained.
- Sometimes service users are more frightened on their first visit to hospital and will need a lot of reassurance and support. In the case of Atul, had that approach described above not succeeded, he would have needed to be assessed for a possible admission under the MHA.

Competing pressures for nurses

If a person does need to come to hospital against their will, the situation is volatile and the person at their most vulnerable. As nurses you may experience competing pressures – on the one hand, paying heed to the person's wishes, creating and maintaining trust and openness, and on the other hand being part of the team that will detain and then keep under detention. So while you wish to have an open and trusting relationship, this can be especially difficult when you are involved in sectioning the person.

Competing interests also arise because of the duty as an employee to follow procedures that may not appear to be the same as best professional practice. This is especially the case with current duties around risk assessments; Trust risk assessment tools can appear over-prescriptive, and be less useful in assessing risk than the exercise of ordinary professional skills (Royal College of Psychiatrists 2009). They can make professionals too risk-averse whereas positive risk-taking can have good results. It can assist a service user to take greater control over their life and their condition, thereby improving their recovery. This is discussed further in Chapter 9.

Challenges and values

The person who has been admitted may be withdrawn and unresponsive, they may be psychotic and experiencing hallucinations; they are likely to be frightened and distressed. They may also be under the influence of alcohol or drugs. Their reasons for objecting to treatment may seem unwise but not necessarily lacking in insight. It is possible that they are angry at their wishes being overridden.

The principles of **respect** and **participation** in the MHA Code of Practice are vital here. Service user surveys consistently report that what most matters is to be listened to in a non-judgemental way, to be kept informed of what is happening, be reassured and involved in decisions about them. They (and you) may find it helpful to have an **Independent Mental Health Advocate** (IMHA) there to help and they may need to have an interpreter. All these may be helpful in their understanding of what is happening and what decisions need to be made. They may also need attention for their physical health – treatment decisions about this are covered by the MCA.

The formal part

As we saw in the Chapter 2, the formal decisions must be taken by specially trained healthcare professionals – psychiatrists, doctors, nurses, AMHPs, ACs and RCs. There are formal roles also for NRs and IMHAs. However, these decisions are taken as part of a multi-disciplinary team and you should be consulted. You may be the person who has spent the most time talking or being with the patient and your impressions and information are essential in the assessment process.

Referral pathways

People come into hospital for assessment and treatment under the MHA by different routes. We have seen the different referral paths of Atul and Sylvia. Let us consider a range of different situations that you may encounter. We return to Joseph, and Genevieve and introduce Lenny and Harun.

- Joseph (see p. 71) has been brought to the hospital as a place of safety for assessment under s.136. He may or may not be admitted as an in-patient depending on the assessment. If he is found to have a **mental disorder** as well as having over-indulged on alcohol, and he meets the other criteria for admission, he may, if he resists, be admitted under the MHA.
- Genevieve (see p. 54) remains under the care of the community mental health team. However, she has not been seen for some weeks. Her neighbours believe she has no food in the house. The electricity supply appears to be cut off. She has been heard shouting at the walls and banging her head. She refuses to open the front door when the community nurse visits her and despite everyone's efforts to persuade her she remains inside. The AMHP seeks a **warrant** from a magistrate to enter the premises and convey her to hospital under **s.135** of the MHA. Returning with the warrant and a police car, the AMHP and psychiatrist open the door, which is not locked, and Genevieve, distressed, agrees to go with them.

- Lenny has a diagnosis of personality disorder and depression. He regularly takes illegal drugs. He was convicted of possession and supply of heroin and of mobile phone theft and was given a prison sentence. In prison he undergoes a drug treatment programme but in the process of the withdrawal phase he becomes seriously depressed and suicidal. He is transferred to a secure hospital for treatment of his mental disorder.
- Harun is receiving a course of **ECT** as an informal patient. He is very weak because he has been eating and drinking very little since his admission to hospital. He wants to leave the hospital now in order to spend the month of Ramadan at the care home with his friend. No doctor is available so the qualified mental health nurse on duty considers it is unsafe for him to leave and she exercises the holding power and he is detained for 6 hours, awaiting the arrival of the doctor who will (if necessary) start the process of detaining Harun.

Steps to take under the MHA

1. Conveying the service user to hospital

> Patients should always be conveyed in the manner which is most likely to preserve their dignity and privacy consistent with managing any risk to their health and safety or to other people.
>
> (MHA Code of Practice 11.2)

The arrival of a police car or an ambulance and a service user's forced exit from their home will be noticed by neighbours and that in itself may be especially upsetting for the service user and experienced as stigmatising. An AMHP and perhaps a doctor or psychiatrist should accompany them to the hospital; and the police may be in attendance if there is a risk to anyone's safety. They may have been transferred for treatment from prison by hospital staff in the prison and the forensic psychiatrist will be involved.

2. Meeting the criteria for admission under the MHA

The **two medical practitioners** need to examine the patient to establish whether the person is suffering from a mental disorder of a **nature or degree that requires treatment in hospital for his or her health or safety or the protection of others**, whether **appropriate treatment** is available and cannot be provided without the person being detained. The AMHP must also be satisfied that the criteria are met and that **detention is appropriate**.

3. Identifying the nearest relative

The NR can be a great support to the service user. There is evidence to suggest that this role is poorly understood by staff and by the person appointed. As a nurse you may be the one who explains the nature of the NR role to family members and to the NR himself or herself. You may also be close enough to the patient to detect if there are problems in that relationship; if, for instance, the patient is unhappy with their NR being involved but is too ill to take an action to have the person displaced, you might need to alert the AMHP to this.

4. Allocating a Responsible Clinician

The RC must keep the patient's situation under review and discharge him or her if the criteria for detention are no longer satisfied. Over time, the situation may change - the patient may, for instance, need to be transferred to another hospital or into the community - or their individual treatment needs may change. In these cases the hospital needs to ensure that there is a transfer of the RC's responsibility to another approved clinician.

5. Making an advocate available

Being part of decision-making processes in hospital is a means for a person to raise their concerns and to take some control over their recovery. However, when a person is mentally ill, their ability to speak up for themselves is impaired. As a nurse you will have the opportunity to help the patient gain access to an advocate who is trained in assisting people to have their voice heard.

The steps to admit a person under the MHA

Scenario: Stephanie

Stephanie is 35. She and her daughter Phoebe, aged 14, live in a council flat. Her mother Martha lives nearby. Stephanie's life has been troubled. She suffered sexual abuse as a child and has undergone therapy to help her deal with this problem. She has difficulty maintaining personal relationships and has been involved in violent incidents with former partners. She has a conviction for assault. She has had several episodes of depression. Because of her problems, her daughter has on several occasions been placed with foster parents as her grandmother Martha has not been considered an appropriate parent on account of her alcohol dependence.

Stephanie is highly intelligent and recently qualified as a financial analyst. She was taken on temporarily at a job in a bank 6 months ago but when her job was not made permanent, she has become very depressed. At times she becomes aggressive and rages against her daughter. Early one morning she is driven to hospital by her friend, Anna, after a serious suicide attempt. When they arrive at hospital she panics and says she does not want to be admitted to the hospital. She curses the nurse who tries to comfort her and becomes very agitated when no one will agree to take her home.

The doctor arranges for her to be assessed by a psychiatrist. The psychiatrist believes that her depression is a **mental disorder** under the MHA. Because of her suicidal behaviours (she was preparing to hang herself), her disorder is of a nature or degree to require assessment or treatment in hospital. It is also the case that the protection of others is involved because her daughter Phoebe is at risk of significant psychological mistreatment. Because she is still objecting to being there, he believes that unless Stephanie changes her mind, treatment will not be able to be given to her without her being detained. He arranges for an AMHP to examine her.

Martha arrives and wants to make an application to section Stephanie herself but the psychiatrist persuades her that it is better for the AMHP to do the application, because she needs to think about the effect this may have on their relationship. Stephanie has been sedated, with her consent, and makes no effort to leave.

In the afternoon the AMHP interviews Stephanie who is now feeling able to take part. On the insistence of her daughter, Martha does not participate in this interview and she leaves the hospital. Anna does join the interview at Stephanie's request. An hour later Martha phones the hospital to say that she found a rope noose in Stephanie's bedroom, confirming what Stephanie said.

The AMHP concludes that Stephanie cannot be treated in the community because she is unsafe and because Martha is unable to take care of her. Being at home would be a risk for her daughter Phoebe. The AMHP identifies Martha formally as the **nearest relative** and informs her of the situation. Stephanie is still insistent that being sectioned in a mental hospital will mean the end of her career. However, the AMHP and psychiatrist believe that the situation is too volatile to allow her to go home so an **emergency application** is made under **s.4.**

The AMHP arranges that Phoebe will stay with foster parents and makes sure that the council flat is secure and that the rent is paid for the month. Later that day a second psychiatrist, Ahmed, assesses Stephanie. He agrees that she should not go home, but considers that she probably has a personality disorder and that she would benefit from dialectical behavioural therapy (DBT). He knows that there is an available therapist, Jemima, who is an **approved clinician** who attends the hospital. Stephanie is detained under **s.2** in order for a full assessment to be done.

After several days the multi-disciplinary team have a **care planning** meeting about Stephanie and talk with her. She is withdrawn and has injured herself by hitting her head on the wall. They conclude that Stephanie remains at risk to herself, that she is likely to have a personality disorder, in addition to depression, and that she needs to be in hospital. The following day there is a new application for an **s.3 treatment** order. The two medical recommendations state that **appropriate treatment** in the form of medication and therapy is available. The AMHP considers that the medication proposed for Stephanie's depression is appropriate treatment. He also believes that therapy, including DBT, is appropriate treatment for her personality disorder. Stephanie is detained under s.3 and Ahmed is appointed **responsible clinician**.

The morning after her admission Stephanie is asked if she will take part in a full assessment of her mental and physical needs. She agrees to this and it is undertaken by the RC and the nurse who has been assigned to her as named nurse. A full record is made in the medical notes.

Her mother Martha will be the nearest relative although Anna knows her needs and circumstances best. Stephanie does not want her mother to have any details of her medical condition. The AMHP might decide that this is a suitable case to apply to the Court for Martha to be displaced.

Stephanie is not qualified to receive the special services of the IMHA until the formal admission process is over. There are, however, other situations which she may need help with immediately after she is detained (e.g. in regard to the NR). If she asks, she should have the chance to phone Peter, the IMHA who has been arranged for her, and to talk privately with him.

Box 7.3 How do the Principles work in selecting an RC?

After some time Stephanie is thriving under the treatment regime being provided by Jemima, the **AC,** and it is Jemima rather than the psychiatrist (who only sees her infrequently) who might be a more suitable RC. On the other hand, Jemima also works in another hospital part-time and the financial resources may not be available to have more of her time allocated to this hospital.

This is adapted from the Code of Practice example.

Purpose principle

- What are Stephanie's main assessment treatment needs?
- Which approved clinician has the expertise to best meet these needs, in order to maximise her well-being and minimise risk of harm to herself or others?

Respect principle

- Does Stephanie have a view about who should be her responsible clinician?
- Is there any reason to think that she would prefer a male rather than a female clinician (or vice versa), or is there a cultural issue to consider in selecting the RC?

Participation principle

- Are there likely to be any difficulties in explaining the options to Stephanie and asking for her view?
- How could these be minimised?
- Should an advocate be involved, and if so, has Stephanie been informed about that? Are there carers, family members or friends whose views ought to be sought and would Stephanie be OK with that?

Effectiveness, efficiency and equity principle

- If Stephanie does have views about a particular professional being allocated as her responsible clinician, and such a clinician is appropriate, is the particular clinician available?
- Could her wishes be accommodated without a disproportionate effect on the clinician's time being available to other patients?

Key points: Summary

- A mental health nurse may have a formal or informal role in the MHA process.
- The named nurse will help the person to understand their rights under the law, check the documentation, do assessments and coordinate with others involved in their care.
- Nurses also have a role in helping a person in crisis feel calmer and more comfortable in the hospital environment.

8 Caring for and treating people in hospital

Learning outcomes

This chapter covers:

- 'Medical treatment' under the MCA and treatment for mental disorder under Part 4 and Part 4A of the MHA (including consent to treatment)
- Human rights and the detained patient
- The role of care planning for those in hospitals

Introduction

In this chapter we consider the legal issues, under the MCA, the MHA and the HRA, when a person covered by those laws is in hospital.

Depending on the kind of hospital you work in, you may be caring for both detained and informal patients. A person may move from being informal to being detained (or the reverse). Their capacity may fluctuate and with it different rules will apply to their treatment. They may lack mental capacity to consent to being in hospital and/or to receiving care and treatment and they may have a physical illness but be detained. All of these factors making legal issues in hospital both complex and important to understand.

Application of the MCA to care and treatment in hospital

In previous chapters we have touched on the application of the MCA to medical treatment and given several examples. You need to use the MCA in determining if a patient has capacity to make decisions about their care and treatment, even if someone is detained under the MHA (although as we discuss below, in most situations covered by Part 4 of the MHA, the person's consent is not required).

The question is whether the person lacks capacity to consent to a particular medical intervention or treatment proposed at a particular time. The assessment may involve members of the multi-disciplinary team and family members and, outside an emergency, would be done as part of the care planning process. However, if you are in charge of the treatment or the examination, you are the one to decide whether or not the person has capacity and if the person lacks capacity, whether giving the treatment can be delayed so the person can make the decision for themselves (e.g. waiting for someone to sober up) and you should consult with others who know the person.

You must provide information about the care or treatment they are being asked to consent to in a way that the person can understand. You must also respect their right to make an unwise decision (e.g. by refusing consent) and not automatically assume that this is proof of a lack of capacity.

There may be differences of opinion as to a patient's capacity – the person may be saying different things to you than to others (maybe in order to please you) or your view may differ from that of the family members. Another opinion (and values-based practice) will be necessary to help resolve these issues.

Scenario: Annie

Annie was admitted to hospital as an informal patient. She has dementia and bowel cancer for which she is being given treatment. She needs to have this monitored by blood tests. She is anxious and resistant when it is mentioned that this will need to occur. Her state of mind and her capacity fluctuate. You need to decide whether she has *capacity to consent* to a blood test. Maybe she has an aversion to needles but a needle phobia would not in itself demonstrate a lack of capacity. You must also not make an assumption about her lack of capacity simply because of her dementia.

If, however, her anxiety affects her judgement so severely that she does lack capacity, you may be able to delay the decision until she is likely to regain capacity. So you find that after Annie has been on home leave for a weekend, her mental state is much better and she is able to understand and appreciate what you are telling her about the blood test.

You need to explain to her clearly and gently the reason for the blood test and the effects of not having it. You should explain any alternative ways of treating her medical problem if she does not agree to blood tests. She may want to have an *advocate* or a family member (if either is available) to help her understand these issues. While this is not a situation in which specialist advocates are provided under either the MHA or the MCA, advocacy services may be available in her hospital. It may help to have the information in writing so she has time to reflect and to discuss it with others helping her before you have a meeting with her.

You make arrangements to discuss it with her after the weekend away, on a morning when she is most alert and in a quiet space. In the discussion it becomes clear that she believes that you are trying to harm her by poisoning her with the injection. You decide she does lack capacity and therefore a *best interests* decision has to be made about whether or not she has the blood test.

You may wish to have an opinion from another member of the clinical team.

Reflective activity

- How would you ascertain Annie's best interests?
- What would be the most salient points to consider?
- Would she be entitled to an IMCA?
- What have you learned from this example?

If the decision is a major or a complex one, you are more likely to need another opinion or a specialist to assess the person's capacity. So, for instance, if Annie is displaying symptoms of dementia and the decision is whether she should move to a different type of residential care or her care needs are to be changed significantly, others will be involved.

Best interests

A determination of **best interests for medical treatment** involves going through all the different steps outlined in the MCA (see Chapter 1 for how to determine a person's best interests). This will include the need to follow decisions made in an **advance decision to refuse treatment (ADRT)**, or by an attorney authorised by a Lasting Power of Attorney, or a court-appointed deputy. You should consult the patient's medical notes where this information should be recorded.

If none of these applies (and this will be the case with the majority of patients), the responsibility will be yours, following the best interests checklist.

Healthcare professionals regularly made 'best interests' decisions about medical treatment before the MCA came into law; it reflects what was already known to be good practice. As one legal case put it, 'best interests' requires examination of

> a broad spectrum of medical, social, emotional and welfare issues [and] . . . the advantages and disadvantages of various treatment and management options, the viability of each such option and its likely effect on the patient and the enjoyment of his or her life. Any likely benefit of the treatment has to be balanced and considered in the light of any additional suffering such treatment might entail.

(Thorpe J re A [2001] 1 FCR 193 at 200)

Of course, it will also be necessary for the decision-maker to go through the list of best interests factors in the MCA.

Planning ahead for care and treatment

As we recall, advance decisions to refuse treatment are a very helpful way for a person to record their wishes about any treatment that they do not wish to be carried out in the future if they lack capacity to consent.

(Re W, Adult: Refusal of Medical Treatment [2002] EWHC 901)

However, if the ADRT is made orally, unless the decision was expressed to a professional and then recorded in the person's notes, it can be hard to establish whether it is valid and applicable. A member of the family may tell you what the patient's expressed wishes were but there could be disagreement on their exact scope or even if the statement was ever made.

Box 8.1 Life-sustaining treatment

Advance decisions to refuse life-sustaining treatment that is necessary for someone who has tried to commit suicide are particularly challenging (e.g. refusing to have a stomach pump after an overdose). They must be in writing and witnessed. If the person was known to have a mental disorder at the time they made an ADRT, it may well be deemed not to be valid and can be over-ruled. However, in one case a person stated that she should not be resuscitated if found in an unconscious state after attempting suicide. The court held that must be respected.

Clearly it is best if an ADRT is in writing. You might wish to encourage a patient leaving hospital to make a written ADRT if they have specific wishes about future treatment they would not want, and they may want it included in their healthcare record. Sometimes people carry a card or bracelet stating their wishes or alerting a hospital to where they have kept an ADRT.

The law says that professionals can stop or withhold treatment because they reasonably believe that a valid and applicable ADRT exists, or they can treat a person because, having tried their best to find out, they do not believe that one exists. If it is an emergency, you can also continue to treat the person if it is necessary to do so, while enquiries are made.

If the ADRT was made a long time ago and has not been updated or reviewed since, then it would be wise to consult people who are close to the person concerned for their views as to whether it can still be said to represent their current wishes.

Scenario: Geoffrey

Geoffrey is 55 and five years ago was admitted to hospital to have treatment for prostate cancer. He was given morphine which made him delirious and distressed. On leaving the hospital he told his wife that he must not be given that again and that he would prefer pain to heavy painkillers like that. 'All of them can make you delirious,' he says. 'I don't want any of them if that situation arises again' (this constitutes a verbal ADRT).

Two years later Geoffrey starts to behave very strangely, including extreme agitation, excitement and grandiose beliefs. This leads to a hospital admission under Section 2 of the MHA where he is diagnosed with bipolar disorder, placed on a Section 3 and forcibly medicated to sedate him. After a few weeks he is much better, recognises that he was unwell and is discharged on oral medication.

Geoffrey decides to make two written ADRTs. One of these is a refusal to be forcibly medicated for his bipolar illness should he be hospitalised again. Part of the ADRT states that he would 'prefer to be placed in seclusion and allowed to calm down naturally'. The second ADRT is a refusal of morphine should he require further treatment for his cancer. Both ADRTs are signed and witnessed by his GP.

Two years later he has another psychiatric episode similar to the first and is admitted to hospital, initially on an informal basis. He lacks capacity to make decisions about treatment and his ADRT for his bipolar illness is respected but he becomes increasingly unwell and is placed on a Section 3. Staff decide to over-rule his ADRT and forcibly medicate him, despite his protests.

While in hospital his cancer flares up again and he requires further treatment. Initially oncology staff want to give him morphine because he is under the MHA but you point out that his ADRT for his cancer cannot be overridden. Staff agree to give him a different analgesic. Unfortunately this has similar side effects to the morphine.

After 6 months in hospital Geoffrey's bipolar illness and cancer have been stabilised and he is discharged. He decides to get legal advice about authorising his wife to make decisions on his behalf about all his medical treatment using a **health and welfare LPA**. The solicitor he consults explains that Geoffrey can do this and this could allow his wife to decide to give or refuse consent about his cancer treatment which would have to be followed by healthcare professionals (even if it involved life-sustaining treatment if Geoffrey wanted to include this), providing she made them in his best interests. She could also do the same for his psychiatric treatment but the solicitor points out that her decisions about his psychiatric treatment can still be overridden if Geoffrey is subject to compulsory treatment in hospital under the MHA. The solicitor explains that to make an LPA, someone like a doctor needs to confirm that Geoffrey understands the purpose of the LPA and that the ADRTs he has made previously would no longer be valid for decisions covered by the LPA.

Reflective activity

What do you think would be the best thing for Geoffrey to do?

Serious medical treatment

As you will recall from Chapter 3, an independent mental health advocate **(IMCA)** must be made available for a person in cases involving 'serious medical treatment' where a person lacking capacity has no family or friends to consult about their best interests. Electro-convulsive therapy (ECT) is a clear example of '**serious medical treatment**' as exemplified in the example of Harun.

Scenario: Harun

Harun is Iraqi. He came to the UK with his son after the Gulf War. He is now 80 years old and has a severe depressive disorder, together with some symptoms of post-traumatic stress disorder. His wife has died and his son Ali has returned to work in Iraq. He is here alone. He was admitted on a previous occasion to hospital and with his consent, underwent ECT, which improved his mood, but left him confused for a short time and maybe has impaired his memory. He lives now in a care home where he initially settled in well and made friends with another resident also from the Arab world. He owns a flat in the town.

Terry, his care coordinator, monitors Harun's mental condition. The symptoms of his illness have worsened and he admits to suicidal thoughts and plans. His care coordinator and the members of the multi-disciplinary team agree that he lacks capacity to make decisions about admission to hospital and treatment because he seems unable to understand that he is ill, and this plan is to help him and not for some form of imprisonment. The team decide that it is in Harun's best interests to be readmitted to hospital for treatment. Harun is admitted to a psychiatric unit as an informal patient. An IMCA, Serge, is appointed because it is likely that 'serious medical treatment' will be proposed and there is no other person to represent Harun's best interests. Serge attends the care meeting bringing with him an interpreter.

The treating psychiatrist proposes a course of ECT. Harun does not either object or agree. Serge seeks to ascertain more clearly how Harun feels about this option. He asks to see the medical records which confirm that Harun is scared of having ECT. He also speaks with the medical team who explain clearly why they consider ECT is on balance in his best interests; the advantages of his mood being much improved outweighing the possible loss of memory or short-term anxiety. Serge explains it very simply to Harun in the presence of the interpreter. He does not resist and seems to accept that this should occur.

Reflective activity

- What have you learned from this example?
- What would happen if Harun then regains capacity to consent?

Medical treatment for mental disorder

People who have capacity

Any person who has capacity to make their own decisions about their medical condition can choose whether or not to take the advice offered by the medical profession – whether it is for tests, observations or medication or other interventions.

A person cannot be given medical treatment unless they *consent* to it after having received the information they need (including about side effects) to make an informed decision. Even if the clinician or a member of the multidisciplinary team disagrees with their decision or considers it unwise or eccentric, the person's decision stands.

In the well-known case of Re B, a woman with capacity asked for the doctors to turn off the ventilator that was keeping her alive. The court ruled, 'A competent patient has an absolute right to refuse to consent to medical treatment for any reason, rational or irrational, or for no reason at all, even when that decision may lead to his or her death' (Re B (Adult: Refusal of Medical Treatment) [2002] 2 All E.R. 449). The machine was turned off and she died.

Box 8.2 What is consent?

A person's consent is to be given to a particular treatment and it should be based on a sufficient knowledge of the purpose, nature, likely effects and risks of that treatment, including whether there are any alternatives to it. It is not possible for a person to make a proper choice if they have not been warned of the risks associated with it (Chester v Asher [2004] UKHL 41).

If you are seeking a person's consent for any intervention or treatment, you should invite questions and answer fully and truthfully. If you are unsure if they have capacity to consent, you must do a mental capacity assessment. People also need to be told that they can withdraw their consent to treatment at any time and should be made aware of what the consequences might be if they do so.

A person who is coerced into taking treatment has not 'consented'. A patient in hospital who gives their consent under the threat from her psychiatrist that they will be sectioned if they do not consent might say that they have not freely consented. Whether or not the person's will is overridden by another is a matter of fact (Freeman v Home Office (No2) [1984] QB 524, CA). The same might be true if a community patient on a CTO was threatened that if he did not consent, he would be recalled and forcibly treated.

Medical Treatment under the Mental Health Act

This topic is extremely complicated. The Care Quality Commission (CQC) has issued guidance for nurses on the administration of medication to patients who are detained in hospital under the MHA and to patients who are subject to SCT in the community and at the point of recall to hospital and revocation of SCT (Care Quality Commission 2012). Mental health nurses should read this guidance in full.

In this chapter we briefly cover treatment for patients detained in hospital and in Chapter 9 we cover treatment for those governed by CTOs.

Box 8.3 When is the patient's consent required under the MHA?

A person who has capacity can only be treated with their consent if they are governed by the following provisions of the MHA. These are people who are:

- held under the holding powers (s.5);
- detained as an emergency (s.5);
- remanded to hospital for reports (s.36);
- detained under the places of safety powers either in conveying the person (s.135);
- placing them in a place of safety (s.136);
- conditionally discharged but restricted (s.41);
- in the community under a community treatment order (s.17A).

A person's consent is required for all treatment for physical disorders as these are outside the MHA.

Part 4 of the MHA: Treatment for mental disorder for detained patients

Under this part of the MHA, **medical treatment for mental disorder** can be given 'by or under the direction of the Approved Clinician' without the detained patient's consent (s.63).

> 'Medical treatment' includes nursing, psychological intervention and specialist mental health habilitation, rehabilitation and care for their mental disorder. It must have a therapeutic purpose – to alleviate or prevent a worsening of, the disorder or one or more of its symptoms or manifestations.
>
> (Section 145(1))

What a 'therapeutic purpose' involves has been extensively tested by case law. In some circumstances simply being in a therapeutic environment of a hospital may even be treatment so long as some specific benefit to the particular individual can be shown. Artificial feeding and hydration (ANH) is accepted as a treatment (including for anorexia nervosa).

For patients who lack capacity, the clinical team must decide what treatment is **appropriate** but it does not have to be in their best interests as it does under the MCA. It may be in order to protect others as well as the patient.

Particularly when a person is in hospital for the first time, has just been admitted or has only newly been diagnosed with a mental disorder, the question of diagnosing and treating their illness will be closely monitored and may need to be adjusted, involving the patient, perhaps family members and the multidisciplinary team. There may be differences of opinion among different clinicians as to the signs and symptoms, and what the underlying diagnosis should be. This can cause anxiety for the patient and as their **named nurse** you should ensure that the person is given the greatest opportunity to participate and as far as possible their wishes and views are respected and acted upon (even though a detained patient can be given treatment without their consent, it is far preferable if they feel able to consent).

Box 8.4 Discussing concerns about treatment choices

Forced treatment with medication is central to the experience of detention. Patients are being forced to take treatments that may ease their suffering and may calm their fears but also may have powerful and distressing side effects. Research shows that the common adverse effects of medication include: serious weight gain leading to obesity (with the associated health risks); sexual problems; diabetes; disabling, embarrassing, and at times painful, movement disorders, disturbance of vision, lethargy and feeling 'drugged-up' all the time (Read 2009). How would this challenge your values-based practice?

Box 8.5 Important note

Capacity to consent to treatment should be under continuous review, especially when a patient has been certified as consenting to treatment by the clinician in charge of his or her treatment.

The patient's medicine card and forms certifying the patient's consent or SOAD certification need to be carefully followed and checked (for instance, if the patient has consented to treatment beyond 3 months, has the appropriate form been completed?). The administration of medicine must also be consistent with Nursing and Midwifery Council (NMC) professional guidance.

A patient may have questions and concerns about their treatment and its side effects. They must be given full information about the alternatives to their treatment and the side effects as would be the case were they not detained.

The CQC reports that patients often showed a limited understanding of their treatment, and say that their doctors have only very briefly discussed it with them (CQC 2011). Patients will also be worried about practical issues about their home, their job, their housing situation, or perhaps their pets. For all these reasons they may also find access to an advocate most helpful and you should then facilitate this. An IMHA can bring an independent voice in helping the patient to understand what treatment is proposed, getting their views on it, articulating their questions and putting forward their opinions.

Treatment for physical disorders

Many people with a serious mental disorder have problems with their physical health as well. This can be associated with socio-economic disadvantage and poor diet. Smoking is higher among this group than among other service users, and those who have taken medication for some time may have become obese or suffer side effects on their internal organs. On admission to hospital it is vital that the person has a rigorous assessment of their physical health and this needs to be monitored during their stay.

Box 8.6 The relationship of mental and physical illness

Mental illness is associated with poor physical health, arising in part from the side effects of medication and an unhealthy lifestyle. It can occur alongside physical illness and can lead to it. Compared with the general population, people with depression are twice as likely to develop type 2 diabetes, three times more likely to have a stroke and five times more likely to have a myocardial infarction. For individuals with schizophrenia, life expectancy is on average 10 years shorter than in the general population. They also experience high rates of obesity, diabetes, osteoporosis and cardiovascular conditions. People with learning disabilities have high levels of physical and mental health needs, in particular in epilepsy, dementia and polypharmacy. Individuals with eating disorders have an increased risk of premature death, skin conditions, gastrointestinal complications, cardiovascular and pulmonary difficulties, osteoporosis and nutritional problems.

(Royal College of Psychiatrists)

Can you be treated under the MHA without consent for your physical disorder?

The answer to this is generally no. However, case law has spelled out exceptions to that general rule; medical treatment under the MHA includes treatment for physical health problems if they arise as a 'cause of consequence' of the mental disorder (B v Croydon [1995] Fam. 133), therefore, investigative procedures are covered.

It is not always straightforward how far this goes. For instance, if the person has been self-harming, their wounds can be treated. Medicine to counteract an overdose is also likely to be covered. In one case the Family Court ordered that an operation for a Caesarean section could go ahead on a detained woman with schizophrenia because it was sufficiently related to the treatment of her mental disorder; particularly as the treatment of antipsychotic drugs could not be resumed until her child was born and for the successful treatment of her schizophrenia, it was necessary for her to give birth to a live child (Tameside & Glossop Acute Care Services Unit v CH [1996] FLR 762).

The special rules (s.57, s.8, s.8A)

The MHA lays down special rules to safeguard the patient when they are receiving more invasive treatments for mental disorders (at present electro-convulsive therapy, psychosurgery, the surgical implant of hormones to reduce the male sex drive) and after they have taken compulsory medication for the mental disorder for 3 months. These rules apply unless the treatment is urgent (see further below).

- *Medication after 3 months*: If the patient refuses to consent or lacks capacity to consent to compulsory medication for their mental disorder, after 3 months from the first treatment it cannot be given any longer without a second opinion approved doctor (SOAD) certifying that the treatment should be given (s.58).
  ECT: Since changes to the law in 2008, an adult with capacity to consent can only be given ECT if they consent. If the person lacks capacity to consent, it requires an SOAD to agree, but if the person lacking capacity has made a valid advance refusal, or where the treatment is refused by a health and welfare attorney or a court or court deputy, it cannot be administered.
  Psychosurgery treatment or the surgical implantation of hormones for the purpose of reducing male sex drive always require the patient to have capacity and to consent AND a statutory second opinion from the SOAD as well.

The rules for this group of interventions apply to informal patients as well as detained ones.

The role of the SOAD and the nurse

The SOAD will examine the patient and see their medical records. They must also consult two other professionals who are involved in their care (one of whom must be a nurse) who should have been professionally concerned with the person's treatment, and have enough knowledge to be helpful to the SOAD. The MHA Code makes clear that if the nurse feels that someone else is better placed to fulfil this role, they should make that known in time for the other person to be selected. The nurse should consider commenting on such matters as:

- the proposed treatment and the person's ability to consent;
- their understanding of the person's views and wishes;
- other treatment options;
- the implications of imposing treatment on a reluctant patient and the reasons why they the patient is refusing treatment.

(MHA Code 24.52)

The nurse should make a record of their consultation with the SOAD to be included in the medical notes.

Section 62 Urgent (emergency) treatment

Section 62 is intended to allow urgent treatment to be given if a SOAD certificate cannot be arranged quickly enough to cope with an emergency. Emergencies cover treatments being immediately necessary:

- to save the patient's life;
- to prevent a serious deterioration in their condition (not being irreversible);
- to alleviate serious suffering (not being irreversible or hazardous);

- or (not being irreversible or hazardous) being the minimum interference necessary to prevent the patient from behaving violently or being a danger to himself or others.

Urgent treatment that is considered necessary under these sections can continue only for as long as it remains immediately necessary. If that is no longer the case, the normal requirements for certificates apply.

If a person who consents to treatment, then withdraws their consent, or loses capacity, or a person without capacity regains their capacity to consent, a new certificate is required. This does not prevent treatment continuing if the AC thinks that stopping it would cause serious suffering to the patient (s.62(2)). It is the responsibility of the nurse administering the prescribed medication to detained patients to ensure that the treatment is authorised.

Let us examine these issues with the scenarios of Joseph, Stephanie and Harun.

Scenario: Joseph (see p. 71)

Joseph has been taken to hospital by the police under s.136. He is admitted under Section 2 for assessment because it is not clear whether he will accept treatment voluntarily or what the treatment plan should be. He is later transferred to an s.3.

It appears that Joseph has a treatment resistant form of schizophrenia. After several months he is still not responding well to the anti-psychotic medication and different combinations of medication are being tried. The RC then decides to try clozapine given that the previous treatments are not proving beneficial. The RC arranges for an SOAD to examine Joseph since it is now 3 months since his first compulsory medication and he is not considered to have capacity to consent. Jennifer, the SOAD, reads Joseph's medical notes and speaks to you about Joseph over the phone. You tell her that you do not believe he has responded well to the medical treatment, that his thinking is still disorganised, and he has paranoid delusions about his mother berating him through the TV set. You know that he is unhappy about taking the clozapine, or any medication that makes him gain weight and affects his sexual functioning and you believe that an alternative drug may be preferable. Joseph believes the drugs are simply being used to control him. You record the conversation in Joseph's notes. The SOAD has an interview with Joseph and also agrees that he continues to lack capacity to make decisions about treatment. She then talks again with the RC and the pharmacist about alternative treatments and then speaks again with Joseph. It is decided to switch to an earlier anti-psychotic drug. Joseph accepts their decision. Jennifer than prepares the certificate stating that Joseph lacks capacity to consent and that the treatment specified is appropriate.

Scenario: Stephanie (see p. 133)

Stephanie wants to discontinue the medication because she does not like the side effects. She believes that it is the therapy that is helping her and it would work better if she were not drugged up. The treating psychiatrist (the AC) disagrees and wants to continue for another few months so Stephanie's condition can be stabilised, and does not believe that the therapy will be as effective if the anti-depressant medication is discontinued.

It is agreed that Stephanie does have capacity to consent, but she is refusing the medication. You mention to the SOAD, Jennifer, that Stephanie might be more agreeable if they were to start on a programme of gradually cutting down the dose with a view to withdrawing from the medication. You think Stephanie finds not being in control as undermining of her self-respect and you believe that if her wishes are ignored, this will exacerbate rather than improve her symptoms. The SOAD listens and, after interviewing Stephanie and consulting the AC, decides to agree with the reduction of the dose. Jennifer prepares the SOAD certificate stating that the treatment (with a lower maximum dose) is appropriate and that Stephanie has capacity to consent but is refusing.

Scenario: Harun (see p. 142)

Harun is detained for treatment under the MHA. Unless he consents, he can now only be given ECT if he continues to lack capacity to make his own decisions. For this reason the SOAD comes to examine Harun. She is given a copy of the treatment plan and looks over the papers. The hospital pharmacist had done a recent review of Harun's medication and her report is included. The SOAD asks to speak with the nurse and has a private discussion with him. She decides that on balance it is not appropriate for Harun to have the ECT at this point but agrees to review the decision after examining him again in a week. On her next visit his condition has deteriorated and she decides that the ECT should go ahead. She specifies the maximum number of treatments that she has authorised.

Reflective activity

- What do you believe is the main protection that the SOAD system gives to the patient?
- What role does the patient's capacity play in decision-making regarding medication?

Care and treatment under the MHA, MCA and human rights issues

Life on the ward

The MCA applies to all decisions for detained patients except those relating specifically to a person's care and treatment for the mental disorder that they have been detained for. All other decisions must follow the principles, processes and safeguards of the MCA.

As we have discussed in Chapters 2 and 3, the Human Rights Act (HRA) and principles of the MHA Code of Practice underpin all practice for detained patients. As nurses working for the NHS – whether in independent or public hospitals – you are directly responsible for complying with the HRA. Articles 2 (the right to life), 3 (freedom from inhuman and degrading treatment), and 8 (the right to private and family life, home and correspondence) are the most relevant.

Management of disturbed behaviour

Patients in hospital for treatment of their mental disorder may present risks to themselves or others because their illness gives rise to disturbed or disruptive behaviour. The law permits any person to restrain another from harming themselves or from harming someone else so long as they only use reasonable and proportionate force (but not for punishment). There are strict rules for using physical restraint, rapid tranquillisation and seclusion. Any of these techniques should only be used when absolutely necessary, and when any other de-escalation techniques have been inadequate.

Seclusion may only be used to contain 'severely disturbed behaviour which is likely to cause harm to others' (MHA Code 15.43) and must be reviewed with an initial multi-disciplinary meeting as soon as possible and after 2 hours by two nurses (or other suitable professionals) – any longer period of seclusion must be reviewed at regular intervals. The MHA Code of Practice sets out clear guidance on all these issues.

Communicating with the outside world

Contact with the outside world is very important, especially for detained patients who are not free to leave the hospital. The right to interfere with a person's mail is very restricted. Communication with others through the telephone, email and the internet should be maintained as far as possible, taking into account the peace and privacy of other patients and any security risks. Privacy in making phone calls should be respected.

The right to receive visitors, including children, is a key element in the person's care and treatment, and prohibiting a visit is a serious interference with this right. It would need discussion within the multi-disciplinary team and a clear justification on grounds of safety, security or the well-being of the patient or others (MHA Code 19.2–19.13). This is not dissimilar to the situation under the DoLS.

Overall, restricting the use of phones, and restrictions on visiting rights may be justifiable for the safety and well-being of the ward but feel also excessive to you and to patients. In all these matters, the MHA Code is the authoritative guide in any individual case and failure to comply with it could be a violation of the patient's human rights.

Other blanket restrictions on detained patients

Detained patients cannot leave the hospital grounds without a formal procedure to give them leave of absence (under s.17). Like other patients, they are not permitted to smoke inside the hospital but, given that they are not free to leave and that their stay may be prolonged, this restriction may affect them more profoundly, unless they can access an open space where smoking is permitted. Patients report being upset and angry with these restrictions and you may need to explain to them the reasons and health benefit for it. Smoking cessation aids should be in place and patients need to be properly supported through the smoking cessation programmes.

A hospital ward where detained patients are living needs to avoid using other blanket security measures that risk restricting them unnecessarily and which might violate their human rights (especially Article 8).

There may be rules restricting access to TV, to fresh air, to food and beverages and to personal effects. In general such rules need to be carefully scrutinised and to be justified for the particular person at the particular time - rather than simply used as blanket rules for everyone. It is understandable that patients who are detained can resent restrictions that feel like punishment for being ill - especially when non-detained patients are not subject to the same degree of control. In some cases, as a person's named nurse, you may want to raise any undue restrictions with your colleagues and negotiate for greater freedom.

Reflective activity

The CQC cites three principles that need to be more carefully observed than they are at present, in some wards: 'least restriction' of patients, 'respect' and 'participation' (CQC 2010). How would these principles apply to a request for a visit from a friend who is known to have taken illicit drugs with the patient? What action would be necessary?

Care planning in hospital

Anyone in hospital for his or her mental disorder has a care plan, under the Care Programme Approach. It will be put together by the multi-disciplinary team together with the patient (and their family member, friend or advocate if they request it). The patient should take as full (and leading) a part as possible in *establishing and reviewing* their plan. Supporting and promoting their equal participation will be part of your role.

The Care Quality Commission reports that where a detained patient is properly involved in their care plan, services will find it easier to meet good practice requirements regarding consent to treatment, and in providing services in the least restrictive manner possible.

> The members of our service user reference panel have told us how important involvement is, what a positive impact it can have on people's experience and their overall feelings about being detained, and how it can help in their journey to recovery.
>
> (CQC 2010)

Box 8.7 A service user's view

The CPA meeting is the patient's meeting. I chose to actually chair my own CPA . . . It really boosted my confidence and I felt extremely involved . . . Within the CPA document, my social worker included my own personal statement and my own personal goals. My parents sat in on all my CPAs, and had the chance to listen and ask questions. They were very proud of me. All in all, I felt everyone was in the picture.

(Member of CQC service user reference panel, CQC 2010, p. 23)

Key points: Summary

- Providing medical treatment to a person is subject to different parts of the law.
- The rules that apply to treatment for both mental and physical illness depend upon whether the person has capacity to make their own decision (unless they are detained under the MHA).
- An advance decision to refuse treatment is an effective way to plan for the future when there are particular treatments that a person would not want to have if they lost capacity to consent.
- For detained patients there are special rules under the MHA under which, with some exceptions, capacity is not relevant. The decision matrix in the Appendix should assist you in dealing with these different circumstances.
- Patients subject to the MHA are a vulnerable group whose human rights need to be safeguarded. The MHA Code of Practice provides useful guidance on this issue.

People leaving hospital

Learning outcomes

This chapter covers:

- The role of the MCA when people leave hospital
- The different processes under the MHA by which a detained person is discharged
  - Tribunal hearings and the roles of staff, including nurses, in that process
  - the importance of care planning in the person's return to community
  - CTOs and how they operate

Introduction

In this chapter we discuss the transition to the community of people who have been detained in hospital under the MHA/DoLS, or who were informal patients but lack the capacity to make all their own decisions about returning to the community. We illustrate these issues through the stories of the service users you have met already.

Taking the steps to return home after an episode of illness in hospital is a time when people are very vulnerable but may need to make complex and varied changes to their previous life. As well as clinicians, a variety of people and services will be involved and their activities will need to be coordinated collaboratively with the service user and their families.

Box 9.1 Definitions: discharge

Discharge has two meanings: an everyday common meaning – (*discharge from hospital* into the community) and a legal meaning under the MHA (*discharge from detention*) or DoLS (*termination of detention*). If a person is discharged from detention they may sometimes remain in hospital as an informal patient particularly where the services they need are not yet in place. When a period of DoLS is *ended*, the authorisation is *terminated*.

In helping a person manage their transition to the community, with all the adjustments that may involve, professionals have duties and wide discretionary powers under mental health law. As nurses, you may not play a formal role as an RC or AC but your knowledge of the service user will be called upon. You will need to assess the service user's capacity for a range of different decisions at different times and to support them in making the decision in question if they lack capacity.

An **informal patient** may leave hospital when they wish, even if it appears to you and others to be an unwise decision. Hospital discharge decisions will often be complex ones – a service user may, for example, have capacity to agree to be discharged but may lack capacity (or need a lot of support to make decisions) about where they are going to live or the care they may need. The process of **values-based practice** may help in situations like these where a number of people (including carers and community mental health team members) are likely to be involved in the decision-making process, with often very different viewpoints.

The MCA and accommodation

A major decision may be about where the person lives; they may have lost their previous accommodation or need somewhere different, given their changed circumstances. This is an important decision for someone who is in an acute care ward and they may need significant support from the mental health team. If the person lacks capacity, a best interests decision must be made.

The MCA (s.38) provides for the appointment of an **IMCA** if the person lacks capacity to make the decision and is going to either a care home or another hospital but only if there is no one else (apart from the professionals caring for them) to consult as to best interests. Patients who were detained under the **DoLS** while in hospital will need a new authorisation if they are returning to a care home or being moved to another hospital and it is thought they will need to be detained there.

Reflective activity

Let's revisit the scenarios of Harun (p. 142), Alice (p. 128) and Atul (p. 116/127). In all cases the question of whether they should return to their old accommodation may arise:

- Should an IMCA be instructed?
- What factors might arise in considering best interests and who should be consulted?

How is a person discharged from detention under the Mental Health Act?

As outlined in Chapter 4, discharging a detained person involves several steps. The process may occur in stages, with possibly:

- **leave of absence**;
- **review of the detention** by hospital managers or a Tribunal;
- becoming a community patient on a **CTO** under the MHA.

Care planning will take place at each stage to prepare for community life.

Leave of absence (s.17 leave)

Leave of absence serves a variety of purposes: to allow a person to keep up their connection with their home and community, to give them some independence (undertaking activities such as shopping or paying bills). In a situation in which others are closely controlling their life, this is one way in which they can take back some autonomy and control. Above all, leave of absence gives the patient and their clinical team a chance to see if they can manage in the community and soon be discharged. Leave can be granted for a temporary period (or series of periods), or for an indefinite time.

They can be permitted to go alone or only with hospital staff, or the RC may put some conditions on their leave (for instance, where they live or where they may go). While it is only the RC who can grant a patient leave of absence, he or she might indicate, for short-term leave, that the exact time can be organised by the nurse or another staff member on the ward.

Let's examine this through the case scenarios of Stephanie and Joseph.

Scenarios: Stephanie and Joseph

Stephanie wants to go shopping. Her RC agrees to a weekly two hours leave of absence to a local shopping centre but stipulates that this would be escorted leave. The nurse in charge of her care arranges the times suitable to the staff and Stephanie. After several successful outings, she is then permitted to go out unescorted. The following month the RC permits her to go home for the weekend without Phoebe and then finally for a weekend with Phoebe. If the leave is for longer than seven days, the law requires the RC to consider whether a CTO would be preferable. In this case the RC decides on shorter trial leave.

In the case of Joseph, the clinical team agrees that he is well enough to leave hospital but it is unclear whether he will continue to take the medication and whether he and Dave could manage a life together while he was still ill. So the RC grants him an extended leave of absence in order to monitor the situation.

The RC needs to ensure that the leave is properly planned, so that the services and accommodation are in place before granting leave. Leave of absence is also required if the patient needs to be treated for their physical condition in another part of the hospital or elsewhere. This may be the case for instance with Sylvia (see p. 128) if her wounds need treatment.

Being discharged from detention – how does it happen?

The RC is the person who formally discharges a detained patient, but the **named nurse** may be the one most aware of how he or she is faring, so will have useful views and information to contribute.

The other avenues for a person to be discharged are:

- a Hospital Managers' Hearing;
- a Tribunal hearing;
- nearest relative discharge.

We shall examine the procedure through the scenario of Harun.

Scenario: Harun

Harun's son Ali arrives in Britain to look after Harun. Ali visits the hospital and Harun wants to leave at once. He says he will be happier with Ali in Harun's flat while a new care home placement can be arranged or arrangements are made for Harun to return to Iraq. As the named nurse, you suggest that Ali discuss Harun's situation with Serge. Serge, who was previously the IMCA, has kept in touch and is now acting as an IMHA for Harun.

Serge suggests applying to the Hospital Managers for a hearing. In this way the RC and others will need to reconsider the legal basis of Harun's detention and justify his continued detention. If that is not successful, Ali might simply use the nearest relative's right to discharge him. You remind Ali that he must give 72 hours' notice to the Hospital Managers so that the RC can decide whether to block the discharge with a 'barring order'.

The Hospital Managers' Hearing takes place in the hospital. The managers ask for reports from the RC, the named nurse and his care coordinator. They have received a copy of the care plan. All the reports state that Harun would be at risk to himself if he was to leave the hospital and that the criteria for detention are still met. The RC opposes the discharge on grounds that the proposed accommodation is not satisfactory for Harun and the managers agree. A member of the managers' panel speaks to Harun and Serge after the hearing to explain the decision more fully.

Although disappointed, Ali then decides to wait until his father's mental state has improved. As Harun continues to improve and requests to go home, Ali gives notice to the Hospital Managers that, in his role as nearest relative, he wishes to discharge Harun. The RC is informed and thinks that Harun would not be 'likely to act in a dangerous manner to him or herself or another person' if discharged. He does not issue a barring order.

Harun's care coordinator holds a care planning meeting during which the question of accommodation is resolved. It is clear that Harun now has capacity to make the decision about where to stay. Despite some misgivings about whether Ali will be able to adequately care for Harun living together in the flat, everyone accepts Harun's decision. The care coordinator sets up an appointment to visit Harun at home and Harun is discharged from hospital the following day.

What have you learned from this scenario?

The Tribunal

The composition and powers of the Tribunal were discussed in Chapter 3. The **medical member** of the Tribunal will examine the patient before the hearing to see if the **criteria for detention** are met. The Tribunal office will have requested written reports from the RC, *a nurse* and the **AMHP**. They must attend the hearing, as their evidence is crucial to the case. The medical member then reports on the interview with the patient. The patient and their lawyer can challenge any of this evidence. An example of an in-patient nursing report is given.

Box 9.2 In-patient nursing report

This report must be up-to-date and specifically prepared for the Tribunal.

In relation to the patient's current in-patient episode, it should include full details of the following:

a the patient's understanding and willingness to accept the current treatment provided or offered for the mental disorder;
b the level of observation to which the patient is subject;
c any occasions on which the patient has been secluded or restrained, including the reasons why seclusion or restraint was considered to be necessary;
d any occasions on which the patient has been absent without leave whilst liable to be detained, or occasions when the patient has failed to return when required, after being granted leave of absence;
e any incidents where the patient has harmed themselves or others, or has threatened other persons with violence.

A copy of the patient's current nursing plan must be appended to the report.

(HM Tribunals Service, *Mental Health Reports*, p. 14)

Let us examine how Tribunals work through the case of Stephanie (see p. 133).

Scenario: Stephanie

Finding a lawyer

Stephanie wants to appeal against her s.3 detention and has asked Nigel, the named nurse, how to do it. Nigel shows her the list of local lawyers, which is kept in the ward. As Stephanie has not used a lawyer in the last 6 months, a new lawyer, Len, can be approached (which Stephanie's IMHA arranges). Len agrees to take the case and contacts the ward in advance to inform them of his visit to Stephanie. At their meeting Len decides that Stephanie has capacity to give him instructions. He advises Stephanie of her legal situation and the likelihood of being discharged. Given that there has been disagreement over her diagnosis and Stephanie is not clear herself which of the diagnoses apply – personality disorder (PD), post-traumatic stress disorder (PTSD), or depression – he requests access to the medical reports and then seeks an independent medical report. He makes the application for discharge and the hospital sends the Tribunal the required reports from Ahmed, the RC, Nigel, and Sally, the AMHP.

Before the Tribunal hearing

A date is set for the hearing to be a month ahead, in the hospital. The day before the hearing, the Tribunal's medical member, Mina, comes to examine Stephanie and she writes her report. Len asks Stephanie if she will attend, advising her that she should try to do so. Stephanie agrees.

The Tribunal hearing

The RC and Nigel and AMHP are all present at the Tribunal hearing. This is important so that they can be questioned on their written reports. The Chairman is a judge who introduces the two other panel members, Mina and Laszlo (the lay member), and speaks to Stephanie. Her mother wishes to attend but as Stephanie objects, so that her nearest relative (her brother) is the only family member to attend.

Mina reports on her interview with Stephanie. In her view and that of the RC, Stephanie still meets the criteria for detention and, because her treatment regime is not settled, her moods remain too unstable to be discharged. Len challenges this, saying that Stephanie feels calmer at home and no longer needs hospital care. There is also a dispute about the medication regime with differing views between the RC (a clinical psychologist) and Stephanie.

The nurse's report includes three examples of Stephanie having threatened violence to other patients and injuries to herself after punching the wall, and the reasons Stephanie gave at the time of these incidents. The report also notes that over the last fortnight no aggressive behaviour has occurred. There is, however, an issue as to whether Stephanie needs to be detained for the protection of others. The nurse's report is accepted by the Tribunal and she is not examined on its contents.

The Tribunal decides that Stephanie should remain detained on s.3. No recommendation is made in relation to a CTO as she is seen as a risk to her daughter.

Reflective activity

This case brings out the need to relate the report to the criteria for detention. Which criteria are relevant to these facts?

Care planning

Leaving the safe environment of a hospital can be a difficult time for a vulnerable person. Things can go wrong if care planning has not been done properly or where services are not joined up or not communicating well. The risk of suicide and self-harm is highest in the first few weeks after discharge from hospital.

Taking the step to resume daily life after an episode of illness involves complex and varied adjustments. Particularly if the hospital stay has been a long one, the service user may need to find new accommodation, their personal relationships may have been damaged (or improved) by the experience, jobs may have been lost or may need to be retained on different terms. Older patients may be transferred back to their care home, or need to find a new one. There may be negotiations with local authorities, housing agencies, social security officers and employers. Further support to become integrated into society may have added challenges for those who have been forensic patients and in prison or secure care for a long period.

For instance, Stephanie will want to rebuild her relationship with her mother and her daughter and try to find work; Joseph will need further rehabilitation and smoking cessation support; Atul will need to continue addressing his drug habit, and drug services will engage with him to that end.

The care planning process

Before someone is discharged from the hospital, whether or not on a CTO, there will be a **care planning meeting** and usually, if there is not yet a care coordinator, one will be appointed. The care coordinator will call the meeting. The patient, the **NR** and **IMHA** (if the patient agrees to them), the RC, nurse and others (e.g. social worker, care home manager, housing support worker) may all attend, depending on who will be involved in working with the service user in the future. If there is to be a new RC in the community for a person on a CTO, they should also be invited.

The CQC: Care planning helps recovery

The need for patients to be able to participate fully in planning their care and treatment applies equally to people on CTOs. We found that people's thoughts about being on a CTO were strongly influenced by whether or not they had been able to participate actively in planning the details of their [CTO]. Those who had were much more likely to view it positively, whereas those who had been less involved tended to see the CTO simply as a mechanism for forcing them to take their medication.

(CQC 2011)

Part of the process will be to decide which services are required as '**aftercare**' under s.117 and who will deliver it.

Aftercare is very broad. It gives people a right to receive health and social care services they need for their mental disorder, and for those services to be free. The service user may need help to establish and maintain their daily living, pay bills, arrange welfare benefits, organise transport, or engage in rehabilitation or education. These matters will be considered in the care planning process. The care plan will name those people and organisations who will be involved in implementing the care plan. The care coordinator is in contact with all the services being provided and they keep an eye on how the arrangements fit together.

Values-based practice and recovery

A key principle of values-based practice is that of promoting recovery. The themes of recovery-based practice will assist you in working positively with the service user and may also lead you to address any of your own attitudes that might reduce the service user's hope and limit their progress.

Useful publications on this include *100 Ways to Support Recovery: A Guide for Mental Health Professionals* by Mike Slade (2009) and *Making Recovery a Reality* by Shepherd et al. (2008).

Box 9.3 Recovery: the key themes

- *Living a life beyond illness* – building a life beyond illness based on self-defined goals not the 'realistic' expectations of professionals [for instance, that employment will be an 'unrealistic' option for Stephanie or Atul].
- *Hope* – believing that one can still pursue one's hopes and aspirations, even with the continuing presence of illness. Not settling for less, i.e. the reduced expectations of others.
- *Agency* – (re)establishing a sense of control over one's life and one's illness by finding personal meaning – an identity which incorporates illness, while retaining a positive sense of self.
- *Opportunity* – to build a life beyond illness using personal strengths and resources, non-mental health agencies, friends and informal supports to achieve real integration in the community.

(Dr Boardman's presentation, CQC Conference, 24 June 2011)

Supervised community treatment/community treatment orders (CTOs)

CTOs have changed practice under the MHA significantly as community teams have begun to take responsibility for operating the MHA in relation to the service users in their care in the community. The proportion of people leaving hospital on a CTO is far higher than expected and in 2011 numbered over 4,000.

It is possible that clinicians use CTOs too readily to be on the safe side in case of relapse; however, the MHA Code of Practice warns against their overuse by stating that the key factor is whether the patient can safely be treated for mental disorder in the community *only* if the responsible clinician retains the **power to recall** the patient to hospital for treatment. The **risk of harm** arising from the patient's disorder and the **likelihood that relapse will occur** are the key factors.

Scenario: Stephanie

Stephanie is persuaded to accept the medication with a view to withdrawing it gradually over the next 6 months. Her condition improves to the point where the multi-disciplinary team decides that she should be discharged from the Section 3.

The issue is whether she should be on a CTO in the community. Her named nurse and RC consider that she does not meet the criteria for a CTO, as it is not necessary that she be subject to the power of recall. She does not have a history of failing to take medication with serious results, nor has she had previous hospital admissions. She does not therefore have a medical history that would indicate the need for a CTO. They both believe that she would undoubtedly resent the intrusion into her life of being on a CTO, find it demoralising to be dictated to, and it would not be therapeutic. Stephanie is now more knowledgeable about her mental health problems and more motivated to take control of her health with ongoing support.

Code of Practice principles

Therefore, applying the principles in the Code of Practice, the **purpose** would not be furthered by a CTO. Instead, the **least restrictive option** and the principles of **respect** for her wishes (she does not want to be on CTO) and **participation** would be satisfied if she was not on a CTO as she would feel more able to work as a partner with the community mental health team in improving her mental state.

Care planning

The main issues to discuss with Stephanie include the situation of Phoebe, Stephanie's employment and her financial affairs. Her mother, Phoebe's foster mother and the local authority Care Protection team are all consulted. Stephanie wants help to mend her relationships with both her mother and her daughter, and hopes that her daughter will eventually come home to live. Having lost confidence in her capacity for employment, she wants to attend a computer skills course and to find work as a volunteer. She is seeking a new claim for welfare benefits and needs help through that process.

The care plan includes these goals and some immediate action. These include enrolling her on a computer course, setting up some family therapy sessions, and arranging for the support worker to help Stephanie arrange her welfare benefits. We might compare this situation with the case of Joseph.

Scenario: Joseph

Joseph is ready to be discharged, to live at home with Dave. After some discussion within the team and then with Joseph, the RC decides that a CTO would be advisable and she contacts Julia who is an AC to suggest that she becomes the new RC. She then explains to Joseph that a CTO is the best way to keep him safe and to ensure that the community mental health team can keep a good eye on his health. It will also mean that they can act quickly if there is a problem with his health deteriorating.

The RC explains that he will be required to continue taking the medication she has prescribed, and that will be put as a condition in the order, together with a requirement that he attends out-patient appointments.

Joseph, very keen to go home, agrees readily with all that is put to him. The RC also speaks to the AMHP, explaining that Joseph can only manage his schizophrenia and stay well if he keeps taking his medication. It appears that the previous relapse that led to his admission was due to his stopping the drugs he was on – here is history that would justify a CTO. She is not satisfied that Joseph understands the full implications of his illness and wants the opportunity to recall him to hospital if necessary. She does not think that any other conditions are necessary – Joseph has a home with his partner, the relationship appears stable and Joseph is not at risk of any misuse of drugs or alcohol. However, she phones Julia who favours a condition that Joseph stays at the same residence. The AMHP agrees with this and with the CTO and Joseph is eventually discharged from hospital.

Some issues to consider in dealing with people on a CTO

1 *Different teams* – Usually, in practice, different teams are responsible for the service user in the community than in hospital and the service user may be transferred to a community somewhere far from where they were in hospital. There may be a new RC and team members. In order to prevent a person being lost in the system, liaison and transfer between the teams is vital.
2 *Conditions generally* – The service user has no right to appeal against the **conditions** stated in the CTO but these should only be imposed after a full discussion with them and their family. It is unlikely to work unless the service user agrees to them. It is not possible for professionals to 'police' the conditions effectively and there is no automatic penalty if the person does not comply, but the RC may decide to amend or remove the condition, or if the person's mental health is also deteriorating, they may recall the person to hospital. Conversely, there might be a reason to discharge the CTO.
3 *The condition to take medical treatment* (see also Chapter 8).

Scenario: Atul

If Atul does not turn up for treatment, what should happen? Clearly his care coordinator would follow up with him and his family. They would seek the reasons why he did not attend and make another appointment for him, preferably at a time of his choosing. If he persistently fails to attend without good reason, and if the treatment regime still is seen as appropriate (other alternatives having been discussed with him and discounted) and if his health deteriorates, his RC and the care coordinator would advise him that a recall to hospital might be necessary.

Conditions raise important issues – when should a person be required to live at a particular address? When should they be prohibited from visiting someone who is seen to constitute a risk for them? The law says that the conditions must relate to the mental disorder and be '**proportionate**' to the risk. What 'proportionate' means in any individual case will require discussion and care, taking into account the principles of the Code of Practice.

To give an example of a condition being offered to a patient, if Atul's drug habit remains a worrying issue, he may accept a condition that he not attend a local club or associate with a particular set of people to protect him from risk. It might even be suggested that he stay away from the local area where drugs are known to be available. Before imposing such a restriction, you would need to show why this was a proportionate response to his risk of taking drugs – it may not be the way Atul had acquired drugs or would be inclined to do so and the level of risk would be too low to justify such a large restriction on his activities.

Box 9.4 Medical treatment of patients on community treatment orders

When a patient is discharged into the community on a CTO, it will include the treatment that the person is to have for their mental disorder. This should have been negotiated with the person prior to their leaving hospital. The following rules apply.

1. A person with capacity cannot be treated without consent even in an emergency. Consent, however, includes consent given or withheld by an attorney authorised by an LPA or deputy authorised by the Court of Protection, or any refusal of consent in a valid and applicable advance decision so long as the person lacks capacity to consent. The person may at any time withdraw that consent if they regain capacity.
2. A person without capacity can be treated if he or she is not actively objecting to treatment or if he or she does object, no force is required, or it is an emergency.
3. Whether or not the person has the capacity to consent, certain treatments can only be given if they have been approved as appropriate with a Part 4A certificate. This is generally required for medication (after the patient has been on supervised community treatment for one month) and for electro-convulsive therapy. An approved clinician prepares the certificate, stating that the person has capacity to consent and has consented.
4. If a patient who has consented to treatment subsequently loses the capacity to do so, a SOAD's Part 4A certificate would be required instead. However, treatment may continue while a certificate is being sought, if the AC thinks that stopping the treatment would cause serious suffering to the patient.

(continued)

5 If the person with capacity withdraws consent, a SOAD certificate is also required. Treatment may not continue against the wishes of a patient who still has capacity to consent, unless the patient was recalled to hospital.
6 Once recalled to hospital, the person is in most respects like a detained patient and treatment without consent can be given.

Recall to hospital

In almost all cases, people on CTOs will have a condition requiring them to take medication (the majority of patients on anti-psychotic medication will be required to have a depot injection at regular intervals). Sometimes they may fail, or refuse, to do so. This is not in itself a ground for **recall to hospital** but may lead to it if the person's health sufficiently deteriorates. If someone on a CTO refuses or fails to have medical treatment for their mental disorder and they have capacity to consent, they can only be given it without their consent if they are recalled to hospital.

However, if the person lacks capacity and cannot consent, it may be best to give the treatment in the community rather than go through what might be an unnecessary process of recalling them to hospital (which could also be distressing). However, the person may not be given treatment if force needs to be used to administer it and if they object to the treatment. Their objection might be evident through their words or behaviour, but if they are not able to communicate clearly, the treatment cannot be given if there is a reason to think that they would object. This should be ascertained by their wishes, feelings, views, beliefs and values (past and present) (MHA Code 23.18).

Treatment cannot be given under a CTO if the person has a valid and applicable **advance decision to refuse the treatment** or an attorney has the authority to withhold consent under an LPA.

The purpose of the recall power is to enable the RC to respond quickly to evidence that the service user's health is deteriorating or they are engaging in high-risk behaviour that relates to their mental disorder. Before the situation becomes critical, the RC can recall the person to hospital. The existence of this power can be seen as both a safety net but also a form of coercion – 'If you do not take your medication and your health declines, I can take you to hospital and treat you any way.' It may be sufficient to monitor the service user's health for a period or they may be content to return to hospital as an informal patient for whatever time is needed to stabilise their condition.

While recall must be to a hospital, treatment may then be given on an outpatient basis. The hospital need not be the patient's responsible hospital (the hospital where the patient was detained immediately before going onto SCT) or under the same management as that hospital. We shall consider this in more detail through looking again at the case of Atul.

Scenario: Atul

Atul complains that he is so drowsy and befuddled that he cannot think clearly enough to even consider finding work and he stops taking the medication. It is apparent to James that Atul has capacity to make this decision – he discusses the side effects clearly and the impact it is having on his life is obvious. His RC, Susan, prescribes another form of anti-psychotic medication. However, his health deteriorates and he begins to experience auditory hallucinations. Susan does a full assessment and concludes that Atul now lacks capacity to decide on whether to take his treatment but it is also clear that he objects to the treatment. Susan recalls him in writing to hospital for 72 hours so that a depot injection can be administered. Atul does not resist this taking place.

At hospital

When Atul arrives at the hospital, he is assessed, given a depot injection and the next steps are discussed within the medical team and with Atul. After 48 hours he does not appear to be suffering from any ill effects from the treatment. It appears to the RC and to the nurse that he is now feeling well enough to return to the community. Atul wants to go home. He would prefer to attend the community clinic regularly for a depot injection rather than continue with oral medication, so the condition on his CTO is changed to reflect that change in his treatment plan.

Two months before the expiry of the CTO, the RC decides that the CTO should be renewed because Atul is benefiting from the degree of supervision that the CTO entails. She consults Susan who agrees. Before submitting a report to the hospital managers, Susan obtains the written agreement of Mary, another AMHP. Mary questions James and Susan as to whether there are sufficient reasons to consider there is a sufficient risk of relapse to Atul's health to justify renewing the CTO. She points out that his family situation is proving a great support to him now and that he has a relationship with a new partner. He is hoping to take up a part-time job at the local supermarket. After some discussion the RC is persuaded that another 6 months on a CTO is unnecessary so long as the community team continue to work with him. The CTO lapses.

What have you learned from this example?

Discharge from a CTO

While a person must be discharged from a CTO once they no longer meet the criteria, in practice, deciding whether the *criteria* are met can be complicated. If the person remains ill, they will usually still meet all the criteria. However, what if they are now managing the treatment well and are able to function adequately? Does this mean that the coercion in the CTO is working, or that the treatment is working (or both)? The critical issue in such a case is whether the RC can justify a need to retain the power of recall. If the person also now appears to accept the need to keep taking treatment, the clinician may be unable to justify it however, a history of relapses or an impending change in circumstances that might threaten their recovery might be reasons. RCs will differ in their professional approach about whether they favour safety and protection over a person's right to autonomy and positive risk-taking. So far, there is no case law to guide them. The Code of Practice principle of respect requires the decision-maker to follow the wishes of each patient wherever. There must be no unlawful discrimination.' So if a person has full capacity and is entitled to take risks with their health, when should clinicians intervene?

As a nurse working with a service user, you will find situations where there is conflicting evidence and conflicting views about the best course to take. Your knowledge of the service user and the goals they have expressed in the care plan will assist you and other members of the community team to resolve these difficulties, with the service user being considered an equal partner in the decisions that are made.

CTOS and forensic patients

CTOs have only been in force since 2008 and in that time there have been few CTOs placed on unrestricted forensic patients as they leave hospital. For forensic patients subject to a restriction order, a CTO is not available. Nevertheless it has been possible under the 1983 MHA to use a form of supervision called *conditional discharge*, which is only available to restricted patients. The Secretary of State can revoke it at any time.

Invariably, conditions are imposed on the patient at the time of discharge. Usual conditions will include residence at a particular address, or as directed by the responsible clinician. Other conditions might be to abstain from illegal drugs or excessive consumption of alcohol, compliance with treatment (albeit on a voluntary basis) and not to contact a victim or victim's family.

In theory, a conditionally discharged patient should not be recalled simply for breaching a condition as, unless in an emergency, there should be up-to-date medical evidence of the person's mental health to justify their recall. Within a month of the return to hospital, the case must be referred to the Tribunal by the Ministry of Justice (s.75).

Scenario: Fred

Fred has a diagnosis of schizophrenia and he has been a regular user of illegal drugs. During a psychotic episode he believed that he was being pursued by demons who were trying to kill him and he attacked a man walking past him with a penknife, in the belief that his own life was in danger. He was found unfit to plead and was transferred to a high security hospital with a restriction order. After three years he was granted a conditional discharge with conditions that he live at the family home, that he take the anti-psychotic medication, that he abstain from illegal drugs and agree to submit to urine

(continued)

tests. If, however, there was evidence that he was taking illegal drugs again, he might be recalled to hospital if the RC also expresses concern to the Ministry of Justice that this is affecting his mental health.

Guardianship

Guardianship is not used very frequently, particularly since the MCA has come into force. In almost all cases it is the local authority that takes on the role of guardian. Some people who have a mental disorder need a guardian, to take charge of their welfare, especially over matters such as their accommodation and their attendance for treatment, for education or for training. Guardianship is most appropriate where the person is likely to respond well to the authority and attention of a guardian and so be more willing to comply with necessary treatment and care. It can be helpful when a person is discharged from hospital, as in the example of Alan.

Scenario: Alan

Alan has an autistic disorder and learning disabilities. He has been unhappy at the home he is in and has been aggressive and disruptive of other residents. He becomes ill and is detained under s.2 for assessment. After 20 days, he is discharged into guardianship so that his accommodation can be monitored. The residential home in which he lives has found him too disruptive and another place needs to be found. It is also important that he continues to attend for therapy and the guardian will ensure that this occurs.

Key points: Summary

- The goal of treatment in hospital should always be to assist the person's recovery so that as soon as possible they can return to their community.
- There are different routes by which discharge can occur and these need careful consideration involving the patient and the clinical team, the AMHP and family or carers.
- The social context and community resources will need to be assessed.
- The decision may be made by the RC, a Tribunal or a Hospital Managers' Hearing.
- The discharge may start with leave of absence and proceed to a CTO, conditional discharge, guardianship or a complete discharge.
- Crucial to the success of any decisions will be a good care plan and the resources available through aftercare, as well as the support the person has in the community to assist them in meeting their own goals for their recovery.

10 Working with people living in care homes

Learning outcomes

This chapter covers:

- Relevant legal principles and process when working with individuals living in care homes
- The importance of supporting people living in care homes to make decisions for themselves
- Why and how decisions may need to be made on behalf of people in care homes who lack capacity to make a decision for themselves
- Deprivation of Liberty Safeguards (DoLS) in care homes
- Scenarios involving people living in care homes who may lack capacity to make decisions for themselves

Introduction

In England and Wales there are between 450,000 and 500,000 people living in residential care (see Box 10.1 for definitions of differ types of care). The majority of these are older people but there are also significant numbers of people with mental health problems and people with learning disabilities living in care homes. The Alzheimer's Society have estimated that two-thirds of all care home residents have some form of dementia, and dementia is the biggest single reason for people over the age of 65 going into a care home.

It is essential that you understand how the Mental Capacity Act (MCA), and the Mental Health Act (MHA) apply in care home settings. It is also essential that you understand how the MCA and the MHA should 'fit' together when you are working with people living in care homes, how the Deprivation of Liberty Safeguards (DoLS) and other relevant legislation, such as the Human Rights Act (HRA) and the Equality Act (EA), apply, and how values-based practice can help when there are difficulties or disagreements. This chapter provides a guide to how this legislation should be applied in practice when working with people living in care homes.

Box 10.1 Definitions: residential care

Care homes provide accommodation for people who cannot live independently or with support in their own home and need assistance with their personal care because of physical and/or mental health problems, learning disabilities or dementia. They are staffed 24 hours a day and all meals are provided. They do not provide 24-hour nursing or medical attention and are therefore defined as social care. People who live in them therefore have to pay for their place or it is paid by their local authority social services if they are unable to pay for themselves.

Care homes with nursing (formerly called *nursing homes*) provide higher levels of care, including qualified nursing care for people who need this because of the severity of their mental or physical disability. Residents require a high level of nursing care and medical attention and these homes are therefore defined as healthcare. The NHS uses these homes for people (mainly older people) who require continuous healthcare treatment (known as 'continuing care') because of a complex, ongoing disability or illness (such as dementia) but do not need to be in hospital to receive this treatment.

Most care homes are run by private or charitable organisations though a few local authorities continue to run care homes themselves. Some NHS trusts have their own facilities for providing 'continuing care', and it can be provided to a person in their own home though this has tended only to be used for people with physical illnesses or disabilities.

Note on terminology: for the purposes of this chapter, the phrase 'care home' will be used to cover both care homes with or without nursing care unless otherwise stated.

As a mental health nurse you may have contact with people with dementia, learning disabilities, or severe mental health problems living in care homes because:

- you are employed to work as a nurse in a care home;
- you are employed to work in another position (e.g. manager) in a care home;
- you work in the community and your caseload includes people living in care homes;
- you work in a hospital and people are admitted from (or discharged to) a care home.

Applying legal principles and values-based practice when working with people living in care homes

In care home settings all the principles of the MCA, the HRA and the Equality Act (EA) apply, together with healthcare ethics, principles contained in the NMC code of conduct, and your organisation's policies and procedures. The MHA may also apply in certain specified situations, such as a compulsory admission into hospital from a care home or discharge from hospital into a care home under certain conditions of the MHA (such as a compulsory treatment order (CTO) or guardianship). Admission and discharge from hospital are described in more detail in Chapters 7 and 9 but where relevant are also referred to in this chapter. It is vital that you also apply the principles of the MHA in any situation involving a person living in a care home who is subject to the MHA. The values and beliefs of the service user, and potentially others involved in their care and support also need to be taken into account. It may feel a bit overwhelming to try and apply all these different principles and values when working as a nurse in a care home, especially if they come into conflict. The values-based practice approach described in Chapter 5 can help you in these situations.

The MCA in care homes

Many people living in care will be able to make a lot of decisions for themselves and, as a nurse, the first principle of the MCA (**assumption of capacity**) is an important starting point for how you work with people. However, for more complex decisions involving care and treatment issues, or where someone's mental health problem, learning disability or dementia is more severe, nurses may need to be more involved in helping someone to make a decision. Giving information in a way that a service user can understand to give or refuse consent to care or treatment that you are responsible for providing, is a key task in virtually any encounter with them. The second principle of the MCA emphasises the importance of **supporting people to make their own decisions**. It is also important to remember that people's choices may be quite unusual or eccentric, or very different to what is considered to be 'normal'. The decisions they make about their lives may not be ones that other people would agree with but this is where the third principle of the MCA is important (**unwise decisions**).

Remember that the MCA applies to big decisions (e.g. what to do with the person's property when they move into a care home, moving into another home, or consent to receiving important treatment) as well as everyday decisions (e.g. if the person needs help to wash themselves or go to the toilet, what clothes the person wants to wear, or what they want to eat). It is vital that you understand how everyday decisions may be just as important in terms of the person's quality of life living in a care home as the big decisions. People living in care homes may not have the mental capacity to make big, complex decisions but are still able to make decisions and express preferences about everyday things.

However, many people in care homes may have difficulty making a decision, despite being given support, about even quite simple aspects of their care or treatment that you are providing to them (e.g. what to wear, what to eat). In these situations it may be necessary to carry out a mental capacity assessment. This must be done in accordance with the MCA. If it shows the person lacks capacity to make the decision, then you can make it in their best interests, in accordance with the fourth and fifth principles of the MCA and (**best interests and less restrictive principles**) the best interests process.

If you follow these principles correctly, then you can legally make the decision or provide care or treatment to the person despite them being unable to give their consent, without fear of being held liable, except where the decisions involves depriving the person of their liberty where extra legal safeguards apply. These are known as the **Deprivation of Liberty Safeguards** (DoLS) and are explained in Chapter 4. Have a look at the Reflective activity to remind yourself about when DoLS should be used in care homes.

Reflective activity: DoLS or the MCA: which to use?

Scenario A: A woman with severe dementia living in a care home occasionally walks out of the home saying she is 'going home to see her mother' but her mother died many years ago and her home has been sold. The care home is well staffed, the woman has a sense of road safety, and never objects when staff gently take her by the arm and guide her back to the care home.

Scenario B: A man with severe learning disabilities living in a care home frequently tries to run out of the home and straight onto a busy road outside the home, showing no awareness of road safety. He is unable to explain why he does this. The home is well staffed but it is not easy to bring him back and at least two members of staff need to regularly physically escort him home. However, he becomes very agitated, is aggressive towards other residents, and has broken windows in order to get out. Interventions that are used with other residents that involve similar behaviour to prevent them from doing this (e.g. distraction with activities they enjoy) do not work and he requires constant staff supervision.

In both scenarios staff in the homes are wondering how best to keep the person safe and whether this can be done under Sections 5 and 6 of the MCA or DoLS.

What do you think is the most appropriate course of action?

It is essential that you also consider other important factors in mental capacity assessments and best interests decisions (Chapter 2 explains these in more detail):

- Be decision-specific and time-specific.
- Not jumping to conclusions because of age, appearance, condition or behaviour.
- Involving others who know the person, and specialists (where necessary).
- Providing the person with practical and appropriate help to be involved in the decision.
- Base your assessment or decision upon a reasonable belief.
- Make a clear recording of your assessment or decision.

You also need to check if the person has a **health and welfare attorney authorised under an LPA**, a **court-appointed deputy**, a **relevant person's representative** (**RPR**), an **advance decision to refuse treatment** (**ADRT**), or is entitled to an IMCA. Remember that an attorney, deputy and ADRT can produce decisions which may be legally binding on nurses even if a nurse disagrees with them.

The MCA and everyday decisions

For many people who need to live in a care home because of an illness such as dementia, their ability to make simple, everyday decisions such as what to wear or to eat, may be extremely limited or fluctuate significantly. This can be challenging for staff because it means they should be constantly assessing a person's capacity and doing as much as they can to support the person to make decisions for themselves, perhaps several times a day. As a nurse you may need to support and advise staff on the importance of doing this and ensure they are able to swiftly undertake simple capacity assessments and making best interests decisions in their work.

It is important also to record this work but clearly it would be very time-consuming and not a good use of resources to record every single capacity assessment and best interests decision. However, ensuring that there are regular staff discussions about individuals' mental capacity and that a record is made whenever there are significant changes in people's ability to make decisions are crucial.

For everyday decisions about the person's care, other staff in the home (including non-nursing staff) should also be aware and able to use the MCA to assess capacity and decide on a person's best interests but you may need to give them advice and guidance about this, especially if they have not received training about the MCA.

Values-based practice and care homes

Although the MCA is critical in how you practise as a nurse working with people living in care homes, you must not lose sight of the other legislation, principles, and ethics of care as outlined in Table 5.1 on page 96. This may at times be challenging because there may be conflicts in your own mind about how to balance up different values, principles or policies, or different and conflicting points of view among those involved. This is where the 'good process' described by values-based practice in Chapter 5 is so important. Unless the situation is an emergency or requires urgent action, then values-based practice provides a framework to resolve these issues.

In situations where there is disagreement, a number of approaches can be taken but the three most advisable ones to use are:

- a team approach to consult with colleagues and staff in the home (although that may be where some of the conflict lies!);
- professional or peer supervision;
- referring the decision to someone with more experience and expertise.

Other approaches could include:

- organising a meeting with all the key players (including the service user and anyone they want to attend with them unless there are very good reasons for not doing this) to try and reach a consensus;
- seeking confidential, external advice, e.g. from the NMC or legal advice;

- contacting the Office of the Public Guardian in situations involving an LPA or court-appointed deputy;
- consulting reliable, good quality guidance and online resources (see Useful resources section).

The MHA and care homes: CTOs, guardianship and Section 17 leave

People living in care homes can be subject to the MHA under a **community treatment order** (**CTO**), **guardianship** or **Section 17 leave** from hospital (see Chapter 9), irrespective of whether they have capacity, providing the criteria of the MHA are met. A person can only be put on a CTO from a **Section 3** or **Section 37** of the MHA when they are in hospital, prior to discharge. A person can be placed on guardianship at any time, whether they are in hospital, the community or a care home. Someone on Section 17 leave still has the legal status of being a hospital patient under the MHA.

A CTO can be overridden if it conflicts with an advance decision to refuse treatment (providing it is valid and applicable to the treatment being given under the CTO), or the decision of an attorney authorised by a health and personal welfare LPA, or the decision of a court-appointed deputy if they have authority to make these decisions. However, care or treatment authorised for someone on Section 17 leave cannot be overridden by an advance decision to refuse treatment or an attorney or deputy even if they relate to the care or treatment being provided. Likewise, an attorney or deputy cannot override a decision made by an MHA guardian about where someone under guardianship should live.

If someone is on a CTO or guardianship, this is a deprivation of liberty but the MHA allows this because it has the appropriate safeguards (representation for the person, right of review and appeal, etc.). However, DoLS can still be used for other aspects of the person's care or treatment which are not covered by the CTO or guardianship, providing the person meets the criteria for the DoLS. For any care or treatment not authorised by the MHA, the MCA continues to apply.

The rest of this chapter follows two scenarios involving using the law with people living in care homes.

Scenario: David (see Chapter 6)

Although David's hospital admission stabilised him for a while and he returned home, his Alzheimer's disease continues to cause a major deterioration in his ability to look after himself. Both you and his care manager are aware of this and it has been confirmed by the paid carer, staff at the day centre, his neighbour Jean, and his daughter Mary. He is much more forgetful, confused, repeatedly says that strangers are coming in and stealing things (though everyone else agrees there is no evidence of this), doesn't wash or eat properly, and on several occasions has left his home and got lost.

Both Mary and the care manager feel that because David is so vulnerable, he needs to be in a residential care home. You remind them that David's capacity to make this decision must be assessed first and then a best interests decision should be made which follows the **best interests checklist** in the MCA – a care home may be in David's best interests but this should not be treated as a foregone conclusion.

Another meeting is held involving David, Mary, the care manager and you at David's house. The aim of the meeting is described to David as 'to help you decide where the best place is for you to live'. Different options are discussed as ways to try and help David understand but apart from saying he is worried about living in his own home and is lonely, he clearly cannot understand or weigh up information, according to the process for **assessing capacity**. You conclude he lacks capacity to make the decision about where to live. Mary is entitled to make the decision for David because of the **LPA** but asks for your assistance to ensure this follows the best interests process correctly. The care home option is explained to David as being a bit like a hotel (he used to like staying in hotels when he was working). David says that he likes the sound of this. It is agreed therefore that he will move into a care home and arrangements are made for this to happen. You remind everyone that there will be lots of other decisions to make as part of this process (e.g. what to do with all David's possessions) and it is important not to assume that David cannot make (or be involved) in these decisions, just because he lacks the capacity to decide about where to live.

A suitable care home nearby is found for David. Mary asks you to help her assess David's capacity to make decisions about his possessions. To do this, you suggest Mary and you take David around his home and get him to point out the things that he really likes or are important and make a list of these. You also ask Mary to make her own list of the things that she thinks are important to David. This helps prioritise and although there are too many things on the lists for David to take with him, it provides a 'short list' to show to David and **support him to make decisions** about wherever possible. Because Mary has authority through the LPA, she makes the decision to sell David's house when he moves into the care home.

David's first few months in the home go well but the Alzheimer's disease continues to cause deterioration in his health. He becomes increasingly confused and can on occasions get agitated and aggressive when staff approach but he doesn't make any attempts to leave the home. However, he has fallen over in the garden and sprained his wrist. Since arriving at the home David has really enjoyed playing cards and board games but always needs someone to do this with.

One day David attempts to leave the care home, saying he wanted to visit his father (who died many years ago). Staff decide he lacks capacity to make this decision and gently restrain him from leaving. David resists for a few minutes but then agrees to stay in the home.

Reflective question

Should staff have obtained a DoLS authorisation to do this or can it be done under Sections 5–6 of the MCA?

Two days later David tries to leave the home again, for the same reason. Again staff restrain him and David agrees to stay. At a staff meeting that you attend it is agreed that if it happens again a member of staff will escort David outside but not leave the grounds of the care home, to see how David responds. When it happens again, this plan is carried out with the member of staff linking arms with David. David wants to walk out of the grounds but gets distracted and forgets the reason why he came out, so agrees to return.

Reflective question

Should staff have obtained a DoLS authorisation to do this or can it be done under Sections 5–6 of the MCA?

However, over the next few months David repeatedly tries to leave the home on a daily basis and there are not always sufficient staff to escort him according to the plan. He becomes agitated when prevented from leaving the home. David has also told Mary when she visits him that he is being 'kept prisoner' and that staff lock him in his room. Although staff reassure Mary this is not the case, Mary becomes more upset and on one occasion accuses staff of mistreating David and threatens to report them to Social Services.

You are asked to attend the next staff meeting where a number of options are discussed including:

- medicating David;
- using distraction techniques;
- changing the security system on the front door;
- restricting Mary's access to David;
- holding a care review meeting involving Mary, Social Services and an IMCA (because of Mary's allegations);
- doing one-to-one supervision with David;
- transferring David to hospital under the MHA;
- getting a DoLS authorisation.

Staff are also worried because Mary's allegation could be reported to the police as evidence of the **MCA criminal offence of ill-treatment or neglect**.

Reflective questions

- What do you think would be the best course of action?
- What are the different values and legal principles that are being expressed through the different options?
- How might differences of opinion be resolved?

(to be continued)

Scenario: Rihanna

Rihanna is a 40-year-old African-Caribbean woman with epilepsy, mild learning disabilities caused by the epilepsy, diabetes and a diagnosis of schizophrenia (for which she receives a fortnightly injection). She lived at home with her mother until her late thirties when she moved into supported accommodation. Rihanna's mother is 73 and suffers from high blood pressure and other physical health problems. Her father died several years ago and her siblings do not have contact with her.

Rihanna is able to make simple decisions about her personal care and everyday tasks and for many years has attended a day centre. Rihanna has had several psychiatric hospital admissions when she has become paranoid and frightened and hits male tenants where she is living. This seems to be linked with times when Rihanna becomes erratic in attending appointment for her anti-psychotic injection. Some of these have been voluntary admissions and others under the MHA.

You are Rihanna's community psychiatric nurse. Rihanna is currently in hospital under **Section 3 of the MHA**. As well as becoming aggressive towards people in the street, the staff at the supported accommodation have been in contact with you saying that they were very worried about Rihanna as she was becoming more aggressive towards them and other tenants as well. She had been neglecting her personal hygiene and refusing to eat properly, resulting in her diabetes worsening, and the number of epileptic seizures has increased. Shortly after the admission, her mother was also admitted to hospital because of her physical health problems.

The admission has helped to calm Rihanna and it has been possible to discuss with Rihanna the reasons for admitting her. However, she has continued to express some anger towards other residents where she has been living, as well as the staff and her mother. She says that she wants to return to where she was living previously, but the staff there are not willing to let this happen because of her aggression and hostility from other tenants. She is ready to be discharged and has been allocated a social worker to assist with this. An assessment of Rihanna's capacity to make decisions about where to live has been undertaken and there is general agreement that her epilepsy has caused a deterioration in her capacity to make decisions. She can no longer retain or use information about where to live and what this involves to make the necessary decisions. It has therefore been agreed that she will move into a care home for people with severe mental illness, in her best interests. This is planned and agreed through a **Section 117** and **Care Programme Approach discharge planning and aftercare meeting**. Rihanna refuses to attend and although her mother is invited, she is too unwell to participate. However, Rihanna is represented by both an **IMHA** and an IMCA to help decide her best interests. The IMCA speaks with Rihanna before the meeting and also visits Rihanna's mother in hospital. She is able to get the mother's views, who agrees that Rihanna should be in a care home. The IMCA points out that Rihanna's mother could have been consulted and therefore it was not an appropriate referral for an IMCA but verbally shares the views of Rihanna and her mother. A care plan is developed and this is explained to Rihanna after the meeting.

Using the values-based practice approach, you and the social worker spend time discussing with Rihanna the move to the care home. You acknowledge that she is not keen to go there but she is also keen to leave hospital. However, her psychiatrist has the view that she will try to leave the home as soon as she moves there because of her behaviour and condition. For these reasons a guardianship or CTO is being considered to convey her and keep her in the home.

Reflective question

Do you think guardianship or a CTO is most appropriate for Rihanna?

Following a visit to the home where Rihanna meets a resident she knows, she changes her mind and agrees to move in there. The move goes smoothly although it is a long way from the day centre so Rihanna stops going there. Before she leaves hospital, she is put on a community treatment order (CTO) to ensure she has her injection (but see Reflective activity box).

Reflective activity: an alternative scenario for Rihanna

Before Rihanna is discharged, a decision is made to take her off the Section 3 so she becomes an informal patient because she is much more settled on the ward. However, she still lacks capacity to consent to being in hospital or agreeing to go to the care home. There are still concerns about taking her to the care home and ensuring she stays there. Several options are available:

- Sections 5 (and 6 if necessary) of the MCA are used to take her to the care home and ensure she stays there.
- If she meets the criteria for the MHA, guardianship could be used to take her to the care home and ensure she stays there.
- DoLS could be used to take her to the care home and ensure she stays there.

Which do you think would be most appropriate?

Three months after Rihanna moves to the home, the staff contact you because they have concerns. They say that Rihanna is dressing inappropriately (she is wandering around the home in her nightdress during the day and night), and sometimes going into other people's rooms and taking money. Staff say that for these reasons they think she lacks capacity and ask you whether they can use DoLS or guardianship to stop her from doing this. You visit Rihanna and meet with her and the home's manager. She tells you that she can't always be bothered to get dressed and goes into other rooms because she is bored, lonely and has no money. You use this conversation to assess her capacity and decide that she has capacity but is making unwise decisions. You discuss this with the manager and point out that under the MCA, appearance and behaviour alone are not reasons for deciding someone lacks capacity. Together, you agree that more effort needs to be put into providing Rihanna with things to do, such as helping with the domestic tasks (which she has said she would like to do) but also that she should be told that the police might be involved if she continues to go into other people's rooms and take money. You emphasise the importance of this being recorded in Rihanna's care plan and communicated to staff. You also suggest that her capacity to make decisions is discussed briefly at the weekly staff meeting so it can be kept under review.

This approach seems to work well for a time but six months later you are contacted again by care home staff who have further concerns. Rihanna has developed a relationship with a new resident who has moved into the home whose name is Mark. Staff tell you that they think the relationship is sexual and because of Rihanna's illnesses do not think it is in her best interests. Again you are asked about DoLS and guardianship. You meet with Rihanna and ask her about the relationship with Mark. It is clear that it is a sexual relationship and it appears that Mark is paying her for sex although Rihanna says that she is consenting to it. It is very difficult to assess whether she has capacity to give her consent because it is a decision that she is making in private with Mark.

You discuss the situation with the manager. There appear to be several options.

If you decide that Rihanna has capacity, should you:

- Do nothing and treat it as an unwise decision?
- Talk to Rihanna and Mark about safe sex?
- Make a referral for a more thorough assessment of capacity to be done?
- Try and supervise the couple more closely to prevent them from having sex?
- Treat it as an adult safeguarding issue and have a meeting, and involve an IMCA or and IMHA?
- Do something else?

If you decide that Rihanna lacks capacity to consent, should you:

- Meet with Mark and Rihanna and explain that it is not in Rihanna's best interests for the sexual relationship to continue?
- Decide that it is in Rihanna's best interests for staff not to interfere?
- Work with Rihanna to improve her understanding so that she has capacity to make a supported decision about whether or not to continue with the sexual relationship?
- Make a referral for a more thorough assessment of capacity to be done?
- Treat it as an adult safeguarding issue and have a meeting, and involve an IMCA or an IMHA?
- Review the conditions of the CTO?

- Use a DoLS to restrict her contact with Mark? If you did this, what restrictions might you use and would she be eligible?
- Move Mark or Rihanna out of the home?
- Call the police and report Mark?
- Do something else?

Scenario: back to David

A multi-disciplinary meeting was held to discuss the situation regarding David, and Mary is invited. You meet with Mary beforehand to explain what the meeting involves and why it is being held. You tell her that a referral has been made to an IMCA (and explain their role) because of the safeguarding concerns that Mary had raised. Mary says she did not report the home but she was very upset, partly about how unwell her father had become. At the meeting the IMCA (who has met with David, Mary and the staff) produces a report stating there is no evidence that David is being kept prisoner or mistreated by the home.

It is agreed at the meeting that two members of staff will spend much more time with David, playing board games with him and supervising him more closely and escorting him outside the home as often as possible. This is recorded in David's care plan and it is agreed that this will be reviewed every week at the staff meeting. The care manager who is also a best interests assessor (BIA) for DoLS says that although this is more restrictive, it does not amount to a deprivation of David's liberty.

The plan works well for a few months but unfortunately David continues to deteriorate. He is constantly trying to leave and is requiring more and more close supervision and restraint by staff which may well be a deprivation of liberty. For these reasons it is decided to make a DoLS application for a standard authorisation.

Reflective questions

- What information and assessments would be needed to demonstrate there is a DoL?
- What role could Mary play and what are her rights?
- What conditions might be attached if a DoLS authorisation was granted?

Key points: Summary

- The MCA is a particularly important law for people living in care homes, many of whom will lack capacity to make decisions. It is always important to support people to make their own decisions about the care they receive even if they cannot make more complex decisions about being in the care home.

- Junior staff may not always be aware of how the MCA applies to the everyday care they provide in care home – as a nurse, it is important you share your knowledge about the MCA and help them to apply it properly.
- The MHA can apply to people in care homes in the form of CTOs, guardianship and Section 17 leave. The MCA applies in different ways depending upon which part of the MHA is being used.
- The MCA can be used to keep people in care homes if they lack capacity to agree to this and it is in their best interests but it is important not to restrict people in ways that contravene their human rights.
- If particular restrictions are required to keep someone in a care home who lacks capacity to agree to this, and it is in their best interests in order to care for them, a DoLS authorisation may be necessary.

11 Working with children and young people

Learning outcomes

This chapter covers:

- The principles and values that apply to work with children and young people
- Special rules that apply to children and young people around capacity or competence to consent to care and treatment
- The application of the Children Act, the MHA and the MCA to children and young people
- Deprivation of liberty under the Children Act 1989

Introduction

Mental ill health among children and young people is a troubling reality. One in ten children between the ages of 5 and 16 has a **mental disorder** (Office for National Statistics 2005). Around 25,000 are admitted to hospital every year because of deliberate self-harm. Nearly 80,000 children and young people suffer from severe depression. A significant majority of children in care and of imprisoned young offenders have a mental disorder.

The National Service Framework for Children, Young People and Maternity Services sets standards for children's health and social services. It aims were to stimulate long-term and sustained improvement in children's health and ensure high quality and integrated health and social care from pregnancy, through to adulthood.

If you are working with children and young people, you will find different and extra issues of law and principle to those for adults, and the law relating to them is complicated. It involves questions of:

- **competence or capacity**;
- the nature and scope of **parental authority**;
- where a child should be accommodated.

These can all be challenging for professionals and families alike.

The MCA and the MHA have specific provisions that apply to this group of people but other legislation, such as the Children Act 1989 and 2004, may apply as well, or instead. Fortunately there is a useful government publication, *The Legal Aspects of the Care and Treatment of Children and Young People with Mental Disorder: A Guide for Professionals* (Department of Health/National Institute for Mental Health in England 2009) which goes through the issues step by step.

In this chapter we consider the relevant law and the issues that may arise when treating a child or young person for mental health problems, whether in the community, hospital or other institutions. Depending on the circumstances, their parents, the local authorities and the courts may also have a role in making decisions on their behalf.

Box 11.1 Definitions

- A child – a person under 16 years of age.
- A young person – a person between 16 and 18 years.
- A 'Gillick' competent child – a child who has the capacity to make the decision in question (so called because of the court case which established the rule, Gillick v. Norfolk and Wisbech Area Health Authority 1986).

Principles and values

The United Nations Convention on the Rights of the Child (UNCRC) is an international treaty to which the UK is a party and therefore is bound to uphold. It contains two core principles:

1. the best interests of the child are a primary consideration in all actions concerning children (Article 3);
2. respect for the views of the child (Article 12) must be 'in a manner consistent with the evolving capacities of the child' (Article 5). As children grow and develop in maturity, their views and wishes should be given greater weight. Their development towards independent adulthood must be respected and promoted.

More detail is spelled out in the MHA Code. All children and young people:

- should always be kept as fully informed as possible;
- should receive clear and detailed information concerning their care and treatment, explained in a way that they can understand and in a format that is accessible to their age;
- have as much right to expect their dignity, privacy and confidentiality to be respected as anyone else;
- should have their views sought and taken into account even where they are assessed as being unable to make a particular decision;
- should have separation from family, carers, friends and community minimised.

The law

Some legislation applies differently depending on the age of the person:

- the MCA does not apply to children but does apply to young people (although the criminal offence applies to people of any age);
- the MHA applies to everyone irrespective of age but also has some special rules for both young people and children;
- DoLS do not apply to children or young people (the Children Act might, however, apply).

The Children Acts apply to everyone under 18 years of age BUT if a child under 17 has long-term needs which are unlikely to be properly met unless the local authority takes parental responsibility for him or her, the local authority may bring care proceedings.

In general, the effect of the above is that a *young person* is presumed capable of making decisions for themselves and their capacity to do so is governed by the MCA. For a *child*, however, it is a question of deciding whether he or she is **Gillick competent**. A second issue is the rights of parents to decide for them or override their wishes.

The following discussion focuses on the rights and powers of children to make their own decision about care and treatment and the legal role played by parents.

Consent to care and treatment: capacity and competence

As the principles stated above demonstrate, children and young people have the same human rights as adults and their views about medical treatment must be respected. If a young person or child needs medical treatment, they must be informed about the treatment, in a manner which is appropriate for their age and maturity. They must have their views listened to. Most importantly, they may have the right to decide whether or not to have the treatment which is proposed. The law on **consent to treatment** for children and young people is complicated and depends on whether the person is consenting or refusing treatment.

People with capacity to consent

Young people are largely considered as adults in so far as consenting to medical treatment is concerned, if they have **capacity**, and their parents' views are not relevant. The rules for determining capacity to consent are the same as for adults. The capacity test is provided in the MCA. The only difference is that a young person is permitted to say that he or she does not feel able to make the required decision. The MCA Code of Practice devotes Chapter 12 to explaining how the law applies to children and young people.

The MHA Code of Practice states 'A young person who has capacity to consent (within the meaning of the MCA) may nonetheless not be capable of consenting, for example, because they are overwhelmed by the implications of the decision' (MHA Code 36.29). Under these circumstances the person with parental responsibility can consent on the young person's behalf.

Children may have the capacity to consent to the treatment, but this will depend on their maturity and the nature or complexity of the treatment, and this will need to be carefully considered on a case-by-case basis. The rule to decide capacity comes from case law and is referred to as the 'Gillick competence' test after the court case that laid down the principle. 'A child has the capacity to reach decisions about medical treatment when she has reached an age where she has sufficient understanding and intelligence to enable her fully to understand what is proposed' (Gillick v. Norfolk and Wisbech Area Health Authority 1986). As with a person who is older, the understanding may fluctuate because of their mental condition, and will need to be monitored, and changes recorded in medical notes. A parent cannot override their child's consent and the child can ask that the treatment be kept confidential.

Box 11.2 Gillick competence: Key points (MHA Code 36.39–36.41)

1 Competence may vary depending on the nature of the decision: The understanding required for different interventions will vary considerably – a child might have competence to consent to some interventions but not others.
2 Competence must be assessed for each decision: the child's competence should be assessed carefully in relation to each decision that needs to be made.
3 Competence may fluctuate: a child may appear to be competent to make a decision on some occasions but other times not be able to do so, for example, where the child's mental disorder is causing his/her mental state to fluctuate significantly. In such cases, consideration should be given to whether the child is truly Gillick competent at any time to take a relevant decision.
4 Before deciding that a child lacks competence, or a young person lacks capacity, to make a particular decision, practitioners should take all practical and appropriate steps to enable the child or young person to make that decision themselves.

What happens if the young person or capable child *refuses* treatment? Can the parent consent on their behalf, overriding their refusal? The MHA Code of Practice states that when a young person is capable but refuses, 'it is not wise to rely on the consent of a person with parental responsibility to treat that person' (MHA Code 36.33). It may be possible for the person to be detained in hospital under the MHA but if the criteria were not met, it would be necessary to get a court order to resolve the matter. In relation to a child, this would also be desirable because the law is still unclear as to whether and when the *zone of parental authority* applies.

People who lack capacity to consent

If a young person lacks capacity to consent due to their mental disorder (i.e. 'an impairment of or disturbance in the functioning of the mind or brain'), the MCA will apply. Parental consent may also be relied upon if the decision is found to be within the zone of parental control. If, however, their lack of capacity arises from immaturity, the MCA does not apply and nor does parental consent. A court order will be needed if treatment is to go ahead.

If the child is not competent to consent, then *the person with parental authority* (usually the parents) can consent on their behalf if it is within the '*zone of parental control*'.

The role of the courts

Although these are the general rules, it is important to note that a court may override the decision of a parent or a child if it is decided that the welfare of the child demands it. This applies even if the child has competence. Either the High Court or the Family Court may be involved.

The role of parents

These rules stated above contain the concepts of parental authority and the zone of parental control.

Box 11.3 Who has parental authority?

- The people with parental authority will usually be the parents. The consent of one parent is sufficient (under Section 2(7) of the Children Act 1989) but both parents and others close to the child should be consulted if possible. This rule is straightforward in most cases but can be problematic if the parents disagree.
- If the parents are separated or divorced, there may be court orders in place and it will be necessary for these to be checked to discover which parent has parental authority.
- If the parents were not married when the child was born, the mother has sole parental authority unless the father, or stepfather, has acquired it by court order, formal agreement or by being registered.
- The local authority may have parental authority if care proceedings have been taken. Decisions about treatment should also be discussed with the parent or other person with parental responsibility unless the local authority has limited their powers.

The local authority

If a child under the age of 17 has long-term needs which are not likely to be met unless the local authority assumes parental responsibility, a care order may be granted to the local authority under the Children Act. It must be shown that the child is suffering or likely to suffer significant harm if an order is not made.

Decisions that are within the zone of parental control

The concept of the zone of parental control derives largely from case law from the European Court of Human Rights. The questions to be asked are:

> Is the decision one that a parent would be expected to make, having regard both to what is considered to be normal practice in our society and to any relevant human rights decisions made by the courts?; and
>
> Are there no indications that the parent might not act in the best interests of the child or young person?
>
> (MHA Code 36.10)

The parameters of the zone will vary from one case to the next: they are determined not only by social norms, but also by the circumstances and dynamics of a specific parent and child or young person. The MHA Code of Practice advises that, in assessing whether a parent's consent may be relied upon as being in the zone of parental control, the following factors might be helpful:

- the nature and invasiveness of what is to be done to the patient (including the extent to which their liberty will be curtailed) – the more extreme the intervention, the more likely it will be that it falls outside the zone;
- whether the patient is resisting – treating a child or young person who is resisting needs more justification;
- the general social standards in force at the time concerning the sorts of decisions it is acceptable for parents to make – anything that goes beyond the kind of decisions parents routinely make will be more suspect;
- the age, maturity and understanding of the child or young person – the greater these are, the more likely it will be that it should be the child or young person who takes the decision; and
- the extent to which a parent's interests may conflict with those of the child or young person – this may suggest that the parent will not act in the child or young person's best interests.

(MHA Code 36.12)

The Mental Health Act 1983

Applying the MHA

The main point to note with the MHA is that, mostly, it applies to people under 18 in the same way as for adults. For example, the child or young person is equally entitled to have access to an advocate although they may need greater help in understanding what that means and what an advocate can do for them; equally they will automatically be assigned a nearest relative if they are detained and they can apply for that person to be displaced as unsuitable for them. They are subject to Part 4 provisions for medical treatment in almost the same way as adults.

So in the rest of this chapter we highlight only where there are differences applying to children and young people.

Admission to hospital under the MHA

- If the young person has capacity, they are treated as an adult and will be admitted as an informal patient if they consent. Section 131 MHA 1983 provides that a young person, who has capacity to make such decisions, cannot have their decision on whether or not to be admitted to hospital overridden by a person with parental responsibility.
- If the young person lacks capacity, there are two options. The MCA applies unless the person needs to be deprived of their liberty. If they do need so, then the MHA will be used unless the criteria are not met, in which case, a court order will be required. Parental consent will be required if the decision falls within the 'zone of parental responsibility' or the MHA if outside the 'zone of parental responsibility'.
- If the child is competent, they can be admitted informally if consenting or with parental consent if refusing and within the 'zone of parental responsibility' (although this is now being challenged by emerging legal opinion that suggests admission to hospital would never be within the zone of parental responsibility or the MHA).
- If the child is incompetent, they can be admitted under parental consent if within the 'zone of parental responsibility' or the MHA.

The process for admitting a person under 18 to hospital under s.2 or s.3 is the same as for adults although one of the MHA assessing team should be trained in CAMHS.

Age-appropriate accommodation

Admitting young people to suitable environments

The MHA places hospital managers under a duty to ensure that patients under 18, whether informal or detained, are (subject to their needs) placed in an environment that is suitable for their age. There is flexibility to allow for any patient under 18 years to be placed on an adult psychiatric ward where his or her needs are better met this way. There is also a new duty (Section 140) on primary care trusts to let local authority social services know where services that can admit young people in an emergency are to be found. The duty also applies to forensic services.

> For the purpose of deciding how to fulfil the duty the managers shall consult a person who appears to them to have knowledge or experience which makes him suitable to be consulted.
>
> (MHA s131A)

So what is taken into account in deciding if the accommodation is appropriate? As the MHA Code spells out, the facilities need to be physically appropriate, the staff need to have the training, skills and knowledge to understand

and address the specific needs of children and young people; the hospital routine should 'allow their personal, social and educational development to continue as normally as possible'; and they need equal access to educational opportunities as their peers, 'to the extent that their mental state makes them able to make use of them' (MHA Code 36.68). For young people approaching 18 years of age, an adult ward may be the most 'suitable' to their needs.

The question whether the environment is suitable will also depend on the nature and severity of the mental disorder, whether they need immediate admission, and the likely length of their stay (for example, whether it is intended to be an interim measure until a more suitable placement can be arranged). In a crisis, the admission of a child or young person onto an adult ward may be suitable because the main priority is providing a safe environment on a temporary basis.

Part 4 Medical treatment

In relation to the special treatments regulated by Part 4 of the MHA the following rules apply.

Electro-convulsive therapy (ECT)

Both detained and informal people under 18s can only be given ECT (except in an emergency):

- If they are capacitous/competent – with their consent and an SOAD certificate.
- If they lack capacity/competence – an application to the court followed (if successful) by an SOAD certificate. It is unlikely that the consent of a parent or guardian will be adequate as being within the zone of parental authority (MHA Code 35.60).

The same rules apply to people on a CTO, except that if they have capacity or competence, they may only be given ECT without consent if they are recalled to hospital.

In a medical emergency the treatment should go ahead as it would for an adult (see Chapter 8).

Appeals against detention

The Hospital Managers must refer the patient to the Tribunal annually, unless the patient has already appealed.

We shall now examine these issues through a series of case scenarios.

Scenario: Sally: use of the MHA

Sally is 15. She has had a difficult relationship with food since she was 10 years old and is now refusing to eat anything other than lettuce and tomatoes, believing she is fat and ugly and that food is poisoning her. She has a poor relationship with her mother. She has had several appointments with a CAMHS psychiatrist in the local community mental health team but missed her last appointment and does not believe she needs to see him again. Her refusal to eat persists and her weight loss continues until she is dangerously thin. Her hair falls out, her skin becomes cracked, her periods cease, and she is always cold and lethargic.

One day, running to school, she collapses with a minor heart attack. She is taken to A&E as an emergency and put on a heart monitor. Later in the day she undergoes a mental health assessment. The decision is made by the psychiatrist, in consultation with her current psychiatrist and her GP and parents, that she needs to be admitted to an in-patient mental health unit. The psychiatrist explains that she has put her body at serious risk. She understands what is being said to her but she does not agree to enter hospital, as she fears that they will make her eat. Her parents are both keen for her to be admitted and her mother is willing to consent on Sally's behalf but the psychiatrist assigned to her care and her named nurse both consider that it is not safe to rely on the mother's consent.

The meeting of the multi-disciplinary team decide that they will need to section Sally under the MHA unless she can be persuaded to remain. Sally remains fearful and intransigent after it is explained to her what is proposed.

The immediate problem is where to place her, as there are no beds in the adolescent unit or in the specialist in-patient unit for eating disorders in a neighbouring hospital. For a short time she will need to stay in an acute adult unit while a suitable longer-term place is found. In the circumstances this would be appropriate accommodation, provided it is temporary.

Sally is eventually admitted to the hospital on a Section 3 after the s.3 procedures are completed and she is put on bed-rest. She is very unhappy being with older women on the ward and is relieved that after two weeks a place is available in a specialist in-patient unit for people with eating disorders where she remains for several months. She is provided with individual and group therapy sessions. She gradually starts to eat small amounts of food again and although her health improves, she remains there for several months.

Reflective activity

- How would Sally's educational needs be met?
- When should she be returned to the community?
- What is the likelihood she would be put on a CTO?
- How would her care be organised in the community?
- Would she continue to have contact with the in-patient psychiatrist?

Scenario: Rekha

Rekha is aged 13. She immigrated from India 5 years ago with her parents and brother. Her father spends most of his time in India on account of his business interests there. She has been recently suffering from symptoms of obsessive compulsive disorder (OCD) that are distressing her. Her compulsion to wash herself so frequently has made her hands chapped and sore and her skin dry and flaking. She has become withdrawn and lonely.

Rekha is taken to a local hospital under s.136 MHA 1983 having been found disturbed and distressed and having slept in the local park after a row with her brother who is impatient with her behaviour. She is then transferred to an adolescent psychiatric unit on the basis of her mother's consent. She repeatedly complains about being in the unit but makes no attempt to walk out.

The multi-disciplinary team, including a psychiatrist with specialty in children and young people, carry out a comprehensive assessment of Rekha and diagnose her as suffering from depression and OCD. They assess her ability to consent to her continuing care and treatment on the unit; if she is able to consent, staff will need to determine that she does consent.

It is decided that she is unable to make decisions at this point owing to her depressed state and the question then arises whether her mother will be able to consent to Rekha's treatment as a decision within the zone of parental control. Her mother's consent can provide sufficient authority to give treatment and care, even if her father does not agree to this (wherever practicable, both parents should be involved in decisions about Rekha's care and treatment but as her father is travelling abroad, this is not practical).

Whether her mother can consent on her behalf involves considerations about the nature of the treatment and care and whether Rekha is resisting this. Although Rekha has said that she wants to leave, she has not made any attempt to do so. When asked for her views about treatment, she has said simply that she hates having to wash herself every five minutes and she will take any pills the doctor gives her. Her treatment, anti-depressant medication, is not intrusive nor will require any form of restraint to administer. Her mother clearly has a deep concern for her daughter and so is likely to be acting in her best interests – therefore it is agreed that the mother can consent on Rekha's behalf.

She is treated with an anti-depressant and a psychologist comes to interview her with a view to treatment for her OCD symptoms. After two weeks she begins to feel a little better and she starts to look at some of her schoolbooks and to watch the TV. When her father visits on his return to the UK, she begs him to let her come home. He wants to discharge her, saying that he plans to take her home for a holiday in Bangladesh during the mid-school term break to visit her grandparents.

There is an immediate meeting of the inter-disciplinary team and the psychiatrist and named nurse have a meeting with Rekha to discuss the proposal and her future care. They are of the view that her OCD symptoms remain severe and she is still depressed. However, she now has capacity to understand the treatment and has sufficient intelligence to do so. She is Gillick competent and can therefore make her own decisions about whether to be in hospital. However, they consider it very unwise for her to travel at this point and think her wish to do so is simply because she wants to go home. Her mother does not oppose her father's wish although she is clearly not happy about it.

The psychiatrist in charge of her treatment decides to do an assessment for her to be detained under the MHA. The main question to decide is whether she needs to remain in hospital or can safely be returned to the community. The MHA Code of Practice says that decisions for a child must involve the least restrictive option and the least interference with her family life.

Reflective activity

- What do you think should be done in this case?
- What extra information might you need in order to decide?

In cases where there is a clear conflict between the parents, rather than relying on the consent of one of the parents, it might be better to detain the child or young person under the MHA 1983 if the criteria are met, or (if the MHA 1983 is not applicable) apply to the court to authorise the care and treatment. (See MHA Code 36.5.) This may be the best course in this case.

The MHA or the Children Act: hospital or secure accommodation?

What if the child or young person needs to be deprived of their liberty in order to treat them or to protect their safety and well-being? There are two options: the MHA or, if they are under 17, the Children Act. Which of these applies depends on the *purpose* for the detention and, therefore, the most appropriate place for them to be placed. If the primary reason is because the person is mentally ill and needs medical treatment in hospital, then the MHA is appropriate.

However, if the main purpose is to provide the child or young person with safety and protection because of their disturbed behaviour, then secure accommodation using Section 25 of the Children Act may be the better choice. It applies when they are likely otherwise to abscond and cause themselves significant harm or if they will injure themselves or another person if they are living elsewhere. S.25 applies to all kinds of secure accommodation from hospitals to care homes but requires a court order if they are locked up for more than 72 hours 'In any event the least restrictive option consistent with the care and treatment objectives for the child should be adopted' (MHA Code 36.18).

Here are two further case scenarios to illustrate this issue. Read them and consider the reflective activity.

Scenario: Rick

Rick is 16 and has a learning disability. He has developed early onset psychosis and has been admitted informally to an adolescent psychiatric unit for assessment and treatment of his mental illness. Rick has settled into the routine, is complying with treatment and his psychotic symptoms have reduced. Although he does not have the capacity to make the decision about his admission to hospital or treatment, he seems content and has not expressed a wish to leave. His parents and community team are in full agreement with his care plan.

Because Rick lacked capacity to decide about his admission to hospital, the legal basis for his informal admission was the MCA. Members of the mental health team and his mother were clear that this was in Rick's best interests, given the severity of his symptoms.

Sometimes Rick walks out of the unit on to a busy road and has put himself at risk because of poor road safety and impulsive behaviour. It is therefore decided that the front door should be kept locked to prevent Rick doing this. Part of Rick's care plan is for staff to support him in going out and teaching him road safety awareness.

Staff raise concerns about whether Rick is in effect being detained and if it is appropriate for him to continue to be cared for on an informal basis. The MCA does not authorise a deprivation of liberty because the DoLS provisions do not apply to those under 18 years and the decision is unlikely to fall within the zone of parental control.

It is clear that Rick's freedom of movement is being restricted. Whether this amounts to a deprivation of liberty will depend upon the particular circumstances. These include the duration of the restriction and whether the care plan allows Rick to leave the unit if accompanied by staff or members of his family. Locking the doors for a few days may be too long. If it is not considered possible to reduce the time when the doors are locked, then consideration should be given to whether Rick's situation meets the criteria for detention under the MHA 1983 or alternatively, whether the High Court may make an order authorising the deprivation of liberty, or whether the situation is so serious as to require secure accommodation under the Children Act.

Scenario: Marcus

Marcus is 14. He is accommodated by Social Services in a children's home as a result of a care order, which has given the local authority parental responsibility. He has suffered from violence and mental abuse from his stepfather directed both to him and to his mother. He has run away several times. His mother has recently moved away from his stepfather and Marcus hopes to begin to re-establish a relationship with her.

He also truants from school and has run away from the children's home on occasions. He abuses illegal drugs and is thought to be working as a child prostitute in order to fund his drug habit. Following police arrest for possession of a small amount of cocaine, he is seen by a psychiatrist and tells her that he intends to kill himself if his life does not improve. He denies that his own behaviour is causing him serious harm and says it is a relief to have some fun, which he will continue to do if he can. He refuses to consider going to hospital. The question that needs to be decided is whether he should be admitted under the MHA.

The forensic nurse and the CAMHS psychiatrist both consider that Marcus is likely to have a mental disorder and should be detained in hospital for assessment under s.2 of the Act and, after the examinations with two medical practitioners and the AMHP, the AMHP makes the application and he is detained.

He is placed in a children's unit in the psychiatric hospital under s.2. After a week, however, it is clear that while he would benefit from being treated with therapy by a child psychiatrist (which he agrees to try) and while Marcus presents a high risk of harm to himself from his reckless behaviour, there is no basis for his being detained for treatment or indeed for remaining in hospital. His main problem is his reckless, dangerous and illegal behaviour.

As a 14-year-old 'child in need' under the care of the local authority, children's services have a role in maintaining Marcus's safety. It is agreed that Marcus needs to be accommodated in a safe environment where he can be helped with his behavioural and psychological problems and his substance abuse can be addressed.

However, his key worker and the team believe it is very likely that Marcus would run away unless he is prevented from doing so. The primary purpose of any intervention will not be to provide treatment but to keep him safe from harm. A suitable place in a youth treatment centre is found for Marcus and after a visit there he agrees to go there but it is clear that he will need to be detained as otherwise he is likely to abscond. The local authority makes an application to the court for a secure accommodation order for 3 months (the longest period allowed).

Reflective activity: Rick and Marcus

Reading through these two scenarios, can you see:

- what legal principles are being employed?
- what acts apply?
- when parental authority is relevant?

Key points: Summary

- The law affecting children and young people depends partly on their age and the nature of the mental health issue. The rights of parents to decide for their children diminish as the child ages.
- The MCA applies to young people and the MHA applies irrespective of age.
- DoLs do not apply and deprivation of liberty may involve the MHA, the Children Act or a court order.
- Special provisions apply to medical treatment for children under the MHA.
- Key concepts to understand include competence, parental authority and the zone of parental control.
- The Children Act has powers to protect children and young people including taking them into care and providing authority for secure accommodation.

Further reading

We have had to deal briefly with the issues in this complex area. In addition to *The Legal Aspects of the Care and Treatment of Children and Young People with Mental Disorder: A Guide for Professionals*, the following sources are also very helpful:

- The RCN Guide, *Mental Health in Children and Young People: An RCN Toolkit for Nurses who Are Not Mental Health Specialists*. It does not cover nursing in CAMHS.
- The Royal College of Psychiatrists website and the Young Minds website contain information for younger and older children, their carers and professionals: http://www.rcpsych.ac.uk/mentalhealthinfo/youngpeople.aspx; http://www.youngminds.org.uk/sfc.

Appendix
Decision matrix for using the MCA, the MHA and DoLS

Table A1 Capacity, consent and compliance: care and treatment in hospital

Key ✓ = can provide care/treatment x = cannot provide care/treatment n/a = not applicable s.5–6 = Sections 5 and 6 of the MCA.

	Has capacity to consent to care/treatment				**Does not have capacity to consent to care/treatment**			
	Care/treatment for mental disorder authorised under the MHA		**Care/treatment for mental or physical disorder not authorised under the MHA**		**Care/treatment for mental disorder authorised under the MHA**		**Care/treatment for mental or physical disorder not authorised under the MHA**	
	Gives consent	**Does not consent**	**Gives consent**	**Does not consent**	**Compliant**	**Non-compliant**	**Compliant**	**Non-compliant**
Informal admission – care/treatment for mental illness/condition	n/a	n/a	✓	x	n/a	n/a	✓ (under s.5 of MCA or DoLS)	n/a (covered by MHA)
Informal admission – other care/treatment	n/a	n/a	✓	x	n/a	n/a	✓ (under s.5 of MCA or DoLS)	✓ (only under MCA s.5–6 or DoLS)
MHA care/treatment for the mental disorder authorised under Part 4[1]	✓	✓	✓	x	✓	✓	✓ (under s.5 of MCA)	✓ (under s.5–6 of MCA)
MHA care/treatment under Part 4 – other care/treatment not authorised by MHA	n/a	n/a	✓	x	n/a	n/a	✓ (only under MCA s.5 <u>not</u> MHA)	✓ (only under MCA s.5–6 <u>not</u> MHA)

(continued)

Table A1 Capacity, consent and compliance: care and treatment in hospital *(continued)*

	Has capacity to consent to care/treatment				**Does not have capacity to consent to care/treatment**			
	Care/treatment for mental disorder authorised under the MHA		**Care/treatment for mental or physical disorder not authorised under the MHA**		**Care/treatment for mental disorder authorised under the MHA**		**Care/treatment for mental or physical disorder not authorised under the MHA**	
	Gives consent	**Does not consent**	**Gives consent**	**Does not consent**	**Compliant**	**Non-compliant**	**Compliant**	**Non-compliant**
MHA care/treatment – ECT	✓	x	n/a	n/a	only if authorised by SOAD (see also Table A.5)	only if authorised by SOAD (see also Table A.5)	n/a	n/a
DoLS apply – care/treatment provided under DoLS	n/a	n/a	n/a	n/a	n/a	n/a	✓	✓
DoLS apply – care/treatment not provided under DoLS	n/a	n/a	n/a	n/a	n/a	n/a	✓ (only under MCA s.5)	✓ (only under MCA s.5–6)

[1]Special rules apply for electro-convulsive therapy (ECT) and neurosurgery, irrespective of whether or not the person is admitted under the MHA. *Neither can be given without the patient's consent* except for ECT provided that a Second Opinion Appointed Doctor (SOAD) has authorised it and there are no MCA refusals or objections (i.e. advance decision to refuse treatment, LPA or deputy objection, or the treatment conflicts with a Court of Protection decision).

Table A2 Capacity, consent and compliance: care and treatment in the community

Key ✓ = can provide care/treatment x = cannot provide care/treatment n/a = not applicable s.5–6 = Sections 5 and 6 of the MCA.

	Has capacity to consent to care/treatment				**Does not have capacity to consent to care/treatment**			
	Care/treatment for mental disorder authorised under the MHA		**Care/treatment for mental or physical disorder not authorised under the MHA**		**Care/treatment for mental disorder authorised under the MHA**		**Care/treatment for mental or physical disorder not authorised under the MHA**	
	Gives consent	**Does not consent**	**Gives consent**	**Does not consent**	**Compliant**	**Non-compliant**	**Compliant**	**Non-compliant**
Not subject to MHA – care/treatment for mental illness/condition	n/a	n/a	✓	x	n/a	n/a	✓ (only under MCA s.5)	✓ (only under MCA s.5–6)
Not subject to MHA – other care/treatment	n/a	n/a	✓	x	n/a	n/a	✓ (only under MCA s.5)	✓ (only under MCA s.5–6)
Community Treatment Order (CTO) – care/treatment authorised by the MHA	✓	x (treatment can only be given in hospital)	✓	x	x (treatment can only be given in hospital)	x (treatment can only be given in hospital)	✓ (only under MCA s.5)	✓ (under MCA s.5–6 or admission under MHA or DoLS)
CTO – other care/treatment not authorised by the MHA	n/a	n/a	✓	x	n/a	n/a	✓ (only under MCA s.5)	✓ (only under MCA s.5–6, or admission under DoLS)

(continued)

Table A2 Capacity, consent and compliance: care and treatment in the community *(continued)*

	Has capacity to consent to care/treatment				Does not have capacity to consent to care/treatment			
	Care/treatment for mental disorder authorised under the MHA		Care/treatment for mental or physical disorder not authorised under the MHA		Care/treatment for mental disorder authorised under the MHA		Care/treatment for mental or physical disorder not authorised under the MHA	
	Gives consent	Does not consent	Gives consent	Does not consent	Compliant	Non-compliant	Compliant	Non-compliant
Guardianship	✓	x (treatment can only be given in hospital)	✓	x	✓	x (treatment can only be given in hospital)	✓ (only under MCA s.5)	✓ (only under MCA s.5–6, or admission under DoLS or MHA)
Section 17 leave – care/treatment authorised by the MHA	✓	✓	✓	x	✓	✓ (but recall to hospital may be more appropriate)	✓ (only under MCA s.5)	✓ (only under MCA s.5–6)
Section 17 leave – other care/treatment not authorised by the MHA	n/a	n/a	✓	x	n/a	n/a	✓ (only under MCA s.5)	✓ (only under MCA s.5–6 or admission under DoLS)

Table A3 Capacity, consent and compliance: care and treatment in care homes

Key ✓ = can provide care/treatment x = cannot provide care/treatment n/a = not applicable s.5–6 = Sections 5 and 6 of the MCA.

	Has capacity to consent to care/treatment				**Does not have capacity to consent to care/treatment**			
	Care/treatment for mental disorder authorised under the MHA		**Care/treatment for mental or physical disorder not authorised under the MHA**		**Care/treatment for mental disorder authorised under the MHA**		**Care/treatment for mental or physical disorder not authorised under the MHA**	
	Gives consent	**Does not consent**	**Gives consent**	**Does not consent**	**Compliant**	**Non-compliant**	**Compliant**	**Non-compliant**
Not subject to MHA or DoLS – care/treatment for mental illness/ condition	n/a	n/a	✓	x	n/a	n/a	✓ (under s.5 of MCA or DoLS)	✓ (only under s.5–6 of MCA, or DoLS, or admission under MHA)
Not subject to MHA or DoLS – other care/ treatment	n/a	n/a	✓	x	n/a	n/a	✓ (under s.5 of MCA or DoLS)	✓ (only under MCA s.5–6 or DoLS)
Community Treatment Order (CTO) – care/ treatment authorised by the MHA	✓	x (treatment can only be given in hospital)	✓	x	x (treatment can only be given in hospital)	x (treatment can only be given in hospital)	✓ (only under MCA s.5)	✓ (under MCA s.5–6 or DoLS, or admission under MHA)
CTO – other care/ treatment not authorised by the MHA	n/a	n/a	✓	x	n/a	n/a	✓ (only under MCA s.5)	✓ (only under MCA s.5–6 or DoLS)

(continued)

Table A3 Capacity, consent and compliance: care and treatment in care homes *(continued)*

	Has capacity to consent to care/treatment				Does not have capacity to consent to care/treatment			
	Care/treatment for mental disorder authorised under the MHA		Care/treatment for mental or physical disorder not authorised under the MHA		Care/treatment for mental disorder authorised under the MHA		Care/treatment for mental or physical disorder not authorised under the MHA	
	Gives consent	Does not consent	Gives consent	Does not consent	Compliant	Non-compliant	Compliant	Non-compliant
Guardianship	✓	× (treatment can only be given in hospital)	✓	×	✓	× (treatment can only be given in hospital)	✓ (only under MCA s.5)	✓ (only under MCA s.5–6 or DoLS, or admission under MHA)
Section 17 leave – care/ treatment authorised by the MHA	✓	✓	✓	×	✓	✓ (but recall to hospital may be more appropriate)	✓ (only under MCA s.5)	✓ (only under MCA s.5–6 or DoLS, or recall to hospital under MHA)
Section 17 leave – other care/treatment not authorised by the MHA	n/a	n/a	✓	×	n/a	n/a	✓ (only under MCA s.5)	✓ (only under MCA s.5–6 or under DoLS)
DoLS apply – care/ treatment provided under DoLS	n/a	n/a	n/a	n/a	n/a	n/a	✓	✓
DoLS apply – care/ treatment not provided under DoLS	n/a	n/a	n/a	n/a	n/a	n/a	✓ (only under MCA s.5)	✓ (only under MCA s.5–6)

Table A4 Capacity, consent and compliance: care and treatment under MHA short-term powers

	Has capacity to consent to care/treatment				**Does not have capacity to consent to care/treatment**			
	Care/treatment for mental disorder authorised under the MHA		**Care/treatment for mental or physical disorder not authorised under the MHA**		**Care/treatment for mental disorder authorised under the MHA**		**Care/treatment for mental or physical disorder not authorised under the MHA**	
	Gives consent	**Does not consent**	**Gives consent**	**Does not consent**	**Compliant**	**Non-compliant**	**Compliant**	**Non-compliant**
MHA admission – care/ treatment for the mental disorder not authorised under Part 4[2]	✓	x	✓	x	n/a	n/a	✓ (under s.5 of MCA	✓ (under s.5–6 of MCA, as an emergency or another MHA section)

[2]The main MHA Sections in this category are short-term Sections e.g. Sections 4, 5, 35, 36, 37, 45A, 135, 136.

Table A5 Advance decisions to refuse treatment (ADRTs), Lasting Power of Attorney (LPAs) and court-appointed deputies: care and treatment in hospital

Key ✓ = can provide care/treatment x = cannot provide care/treatment if ADRT, LPA or deputy does not permit/consent n/a = not applicable.

	Advance decision to refuse treatment involving:		**Health and welfare LPA with authority to refuse consent to:**		**Court-appointed deputy with authority to refuse consent to:**	
	Care/treatment for mental disorder authorised under the MHA	**Care/treatment for mental or physical disorder not authorised under the MHA**	**Care/treatment for mental disorder authorised under the MHA**	**Care/treatment for mental or physical disorder not authorised under the MHA**	**Care/treatment for mental disorder authorised under the MHA**	**Care/treatment for mental or physical disorder not authorised under the MHA**
Informal admission – care/treatment for mental illness/condition	n/a	x	n/a	x	n/a	x
Informal admission – other care/treatment	n/a	x	n/a	x	n/a	x
MHA care/treatment for the mental disorder authorised under Part 4[3]	✓	x	✓	x	✓	x
MHA care/treatment under Part 4 – other care/treatment not authorised by MHA	n/a	x	n/a	x	n/a	x
MHA care/treatment – ECT	x	n/a	x	n/a	x	n/a

(continued)

Table A5 Advance decisions to refuse treatment (ADRTs), Lasting Power of Attorney (LPAs) and court-appointed deputies: care and treatment in hospital (*continued*)

	Advance decision to refuse treatment involving:		**Health and welfare LPA with authority to refuse consent to:**		**Court-appointed deputy with authority to refuse consent to:**	
	Care/treatment for mental disorder authorised under the MHA	**Care/treatment for mental or physical disorder not authorised under the MHA**	**Care/treatment for mental disorder authorised under the MHA**	**Care/treatment for mental or physical disorder not authorised under the MHA**	**Care/treatment for mental disorder authorised under the MHA**	**Care/treatment for mental or physical disorder not authorised under the MHA**
DoLS (standard authorisation) apply – any care/treatment	n/a	x	n/a	x	n/a	x
DoLS (urgent authorisation) apply – care/treatment authorised under DoLS	n/a	✓	n/a	✓	n/a	✓
DoLS (urgent authorisation) apply – care/treatment not authorised under DoLS	n/a	x	n/a	x	n/a	x

[3]Special rules apply for electro-convulsive therapy (ECT) and neurosurgery, irrespective of whether or not the person is admitted under the MHA. *Neither can be given without the patient's consent* except for ECT provided that a Second Opinion Appointed Doctor (SOAD) has authorised it and there are no MCA refusals or objections (i.e. advance decision to refuse treatment, LPA or deputy objection, or the treatment conflicts with a Court of Protection decision).

Note: The same criteria apply even if ADRT/LPA involves life-sustaining treatment providing the ADRT covers this correctly, or the LPA authorises the attorney to make this decision and it is the person's best interests. See also note above regarding neurosurgery and ECT.

Table A6 ADRTs, LPAs and court-appointed deputies: care and treatment in the community

Key ✓ = can provide care/treatment x = cannot provide care/treatment if ADRT, LPA or deputy does not permit/consent n/a = not applicable.

	Advance decision to refuse treatment involving		**Health and welfare LPA with authority to refuse consent**		**Court-appointed deputy with authority to refuse consent**	
	Care/treatment for mental disorder authorised under the MHA	**Care/treatment for mental or physical disorder not authorised under the MHA**	**Care/treatment for mental disorder authorised under the MHA**	**Care/treatment for mental or physical disorder not authorised under the MHA**	**Care/treatment for mental disorder authorised under the MHA**	**Care/treatment for mental or physical disorder not authorised under the MHA**
Not subject to MHA – care/treatment for mental health	n/a	x	n/a	x	n/a	x
Not subject to MHA – other care/treatment	n/a	x	n/a	x	n/a	x
Community Treatment Order – care/ treatment for mental disorder	x	x	x	x	x	x
Community Treatment Order – other care/ treatment	n/a	x	n/a	x	n/a	x
Guardianship (guardian's powers only)	n/a	x	✓	x	✓	x

(continued)

Table A6 ADRTs, LPAs and court-appointed deputies: care and treatment in the community (*continued*)

	Advance decision to refuse treatment involving		**Health and welfare LPA with authority to refuse consent**		**Court-appointed deputy with authority to refuse consent**	
	Care/treatment for mental disorder authorised under the MHA	**Care/treatment for mental or physical disorder not authorised under the MHA**	**Care/treatment for mental disorder authorised under the MHA**	**Care/treatment for mental or physical disorder not authorised under the MHA**	**Care/treatment for mental disorder authorised under the MHA**	**Care/treatment for mental or physical disorder not authorised under the MHA**
Section 17 leave – care/treatment authorised by the MHA	✓	x	✓	x	✓	x
Section 17 leave – other care/treatment not authorised by the MHA	n/a	x	n/a	x	n/a	x

Note: Same criteria apply even if ADRT/LPA involves life-sustaining treatment providing the ADRT covers this correctly, or the LPA authorises the attorney to make this decision and it is the person's best interests.

Table A7 ADRTs, LPAs and court-appointed deputies: care and treatment in care homes

Key ✓ = can provide care/treatment x = cannot provide care/treatment if ADRT, LPA or deputy does not permit/consent n/a = not applicable.

	Advance decision to refuse treatment involving		**Health and welfare LPA with authority to refuse consent to**		**Court-appointed deputy with authority to refuse consent to**	
	Care/treatment for mental disorder authorised under the MHA	**Care/treatment for mental or physical disorder not authorised under the MHA**	**Care/treatment for mental disorder authorised under the MHA**	**Care/treatment for mental or physical disorder not authorised under the MHA**	**Care/treatment for mental disorder authorised under the MHA**	**Care/treatment for mental or physical disorder not authorised under the MHA**
Not subject to MHA or DoLS – care/treatment for mental illness/condition	n/a	x	n/a	x	n/a	x
Not subject to MHA or DoLS – other care/treatment	n/a	x	n/a	x	n/a	x
Community Treatment Order – care/treatment for mental disorder	x	x	x	x	x	x
Community Treatment Order – other care/treatment	n/a	x	n/a	x	n/a	x
Guardianship (guardian's powers only)	n/a	x	✓	x	✓	x
Section 17 leave – care/treatment authorised by the MHA	✓	x	✓	x	✓	x

(continued)

Table A7 ADRTs, LPAs and court-appointed deputies: care and treatment in care homes (*continued*)

	Advance decision to refuse treatment involving		Health and welfare LPA with authority to refuse consent to		Court-appointed deputy with authority to refuse consent to	
	Care/treatment for mental disorder authorised under the MHA	Care/treatment for mental or physical disorder not authorised under the MHA	Care/treatment for mental disorder authorised under the MHA	Care/treatment for mental or physical disorder not authorised under the MHA	Care/treatment for mental disorder authorised under the MHA	Care/treatment for mental or physical disorder not authorised under the MHA
Section 17 leave – other care/treatment not authorised by the MHA	n/a	x	n/a	x	n/a	x
DoLS (standard authorisation) apply – any care/treatment	n/a	x	n/a	x	n/a	x
DoLS (urgent authorisation) apply – care/treatment authorised under DoLS	n/a	✓	n/a	✓	n/a	✓
DoLS (urgent authorisation) apply – care/treatment not authorised under DoLS	n/a	x	n/a	x	n/a	x

Note for Table A7: Same criteria apply wherever the person may be even if ADRT/LPA involve the refusal of consent to the provision or continuation of life-sustaining treatment, providing the ADRT applies to this treatment and is valid and applicable, or the LPA authorises the attorney to make this decision and it is the person's best interests.

Notes for Tables A5–7: Court-appointed deputies cannot refuse consent for life-sustaining treatment – only the Court can make these decisions.

ADRTs, LPAs, deputies – which/who has priority?

- An ADRT made after an LPA cannot be overridden by the attorney.
- An ADRT cannot be overridden by a court-appointed deputy.
- An attorney can override an ADRT if the LPA was made after the ADRT and gives the attorney the authority to make decisions about the same treatment.
- An attorney's decision cannot be overridden by a court-appointed deputy if the attorney was appointed first.

Useful resources

- **The Alzheimer's Society** – the leading dementia charity and has useful online factsheets on the MCA and MHA: http://www.alzheimers.org.uk/factsheets.
- **The Care Quality Commission (CQC)** – monitors and publishes reports on the Mental Health Act and Deprivation of Liberty Safeguards (and the MCA):
  - General information for mental health services: http://www.cqc.org.uk/organisations-we-regulate/mental-health-services,
  - Mental Health Act 1983: http://www.cqc.org.uk/public/what-are-standards/your-rights-under-mental-health-act,
  - DoLS (and MCA): http://www.cqc.org.uk/organisations-we-regulate/registered-services/guidance-about-compliance/how-mental-capacity-act-2005.
- **The Centre for Mental Health** – a national mental health research and development charity – www.centreformentalhealth.org.uk.
- **The Department of Health** – practitioner information and training materials:
  - Mental Capacity Act 2005 Code of Practice: http://webarchive.nationalarchives.gov.uk/20110907114137/http://www.justice.gov.uk/guidance/protecting-the-vulnerable/mental-capacity-act/index.htm;
  - Deprivation of Liberty Safeguards Code of Practice: http://www.dh.gov.uk/en/Publicationsandstatistics/Publications/PublicationsPolicyAndGuidance/DH_085476;
  - Mental Health Act 1983 Code of Practice: http://www.dh.gov.uk/en/Publicationsandstatistics/Publications/PublicationsPolicyAndGuidance/DH_084597;
  - MCA training materials: http://www.dh.gov.uk/en/Publicationsandstatistics/Publications/PublicationsPolicyAndGuidance/DH_074491.
  - MHA training materials: http://www.nmhdu.org.uk/our-work/improving-mental-health-care-pathways/implementing-the-amended-mental-health-act-1983/training.
- **The Equality and Human Rights Commission (ECHR)** – the statutory body that deals with human rights and equality issues. It provides information about HRA, EA and CRPD, including a helpline. More details at: www.equalityhumanrights.co.
- **Mencap** – the leading learning disabilities charity – http://www.mencap.org.uk/.
- **Mental Capacity Community of Practice** – an online national community to share information, good practice, policies and procedures related to the Mental Capacity Act and Deprivation of Liberty Safeguards: http://www.communities.idea.gov.uk/comm/landing-home.do?id=8606690.
- **Mental Health Care** – online information about the Mental Health Act produced by the Institute of Psychiatry, Rethink, and the South London and

Maudsley NHS Foundation Trust: http://www.mentalhealthcare.org.uk/mental_health_act.

- **The Mental Health Foundation** – the leading UK research and development charity for mental health, dementia and learning disabilities and provides free online mental capacity resources for assessing capacity (AMCAT) and making best interests decisions: www.mentalhealth.org.uk:
  - assessing capacity: www.amcat.org.uk
  - best interests decisions: www.bestinterests.org.uk.
- **Mind** – the leading mental health charity provides information and guidance about the MHA and MCA and has useful online information about the MCA and MHA: http://www.mind.org.uk/help/information_and_advice.
- **The National Institute for Health and Clinical Excellence (NICE)** – provides information and guidance about appropriate care and treatment: http://www.nice.org.uk/.
- **The Nursing and Midwifery Council (NMC)** – information on the MCA: http://www.nmc-uk.org/Nurses-and-midwives/Advice-by-topic/A/Advice/Mental-Capacity-Act-2005/.
- **The Office of the Public Guardian (OPG)**: http://www.justice.gov.uk/about/opg.
- **The Royal College of Nursing (RCN)** – the nurses' professional body. The RCN supports a mental health forum: http://www.rcn.org.uk/development/communities/rcn_forum_communities/mental_health.
- **The Royal College of Psychiatrists** – psychiatrists' professional body: provides briefings, reports, professional and service user guidance and research evidence on mental health, medical treatments, as well as dementia and learning disabilities: www.rcpsych.ac.uk.
- **The Social Care Institute for Excellence (SCIE)** – provides information and guidance about appropriate care and has extensive resources about mental capacity resources (especially useful for working with people in the community and care homes): http://www.scie.org.uk/topic/careneeds/mentalcapacity.
- **The Welsh Assembly Government** – responsible for implementing the MCA in Wales including commissioning IMCA services: http://wales.gov.uk/topics/health/nhswales/healthservice/mentalhealthservices/mentalcapacityact/?lang=en.

Further reading

Bowen, P. (2007). *The Mental Health Act 2007.* Oxford: Oxford University Press. A full account of the Mental Health Act 1983 as amended by the Mental Health Act 2007 and the Mental Capacity Act 2005.

Fennell, P. (2007) *Mental Health: Law and Practice.* Bristol: Jordans. A full account of the Mental Health Act 1983 as amended by the Mental Health Act 2007.

Hale, B. (2010) *Mental Health Law*, 5th edn. London: Sweet and Maxwell.

Jones, R.M. (2008) *Mental Health Act Manual*, (2th edn. London: Sweet and Maxwell. The Mental Health Act 1983 as amended by the 2007 Act and the accompanying rules, regulations and Code of Practice.

Maden, A. and Spencer-Lane, T. (2010). *Essential Mental Health Law.* London: Hammersmith Press. A brief guide to the Mental Health Act 1983 as amended by the Mental Health Act 2007 and the Mental Capacity Act 2005.

Mental Health Foundation (2012) *Mental Capacity and the Mental Capacity Act 2005: A Literature Review.* London: Mental Health Foundation. A useful overview of mental capacity research.

National Mental Health Development Unit (2009) *The Legal Aspects of the Care and Treatment of Children and Young People with Mental Disorder: A Guide for Professionals*. Available at: http://www.nmhdu.org.uk/silo/files/the-legal-aspects-of-the-care-and-treatment-of-children-and-young-people.pdf.

Norman, I. and Ryrie, I. (2009) *The Art and Science of Mental Health Nursing.* Maidenhead: Open University Press.

Nursing and Midwifery Council (2008) *Code of Professional Conduct.* London: NMC.

South London and Maudsley NHS Foundation Trust (2010) *The Maze: A Practical Guide to the Mental Health Act 1983*. London: DH.

Woodbridge, K. and Fulford, B. (2004) *Whose Values?* London: Centre for Mental Health. A workbook for values-based practice in mental health.

Bibliography

Alzheimer's Society (2010) *My Name Is Not Dementia*. London: The Alzheimer's Society.

Barker, P. (2009) *Psychiatric and Mental Health Nursing: The Craft of Caring*. London: Hodder Arnold.

Bowen, P. (2007) *The Mental Health Act 2007*. Oxford: Oxford University Press.

Care Quality Commission (2010) *Monitoring the Use of the Mental Health Act in 2009/10*. Available at: http://www.cqc.org.uk/sites/default/files/media/documents/cqc_mha_report_2011_main_final.pdf/.

Care Quality Commission (2011) *Annual Report*. London: CQC.

Care Quality Commission (2012) *Nurses, the Administration of Medicine for Mental Disorder and the Mental Health Act 1983*. Available at: http://www.cqc.org.uk/sites/default/files/media/documents/20100101_11_nurses__the_administration_of_medicine_for_mental_disorder.pdf.

Churchill, R., Owen, G., Singh, S., Hotopf, M., (2007) *International Experiences of Using Community Treatment Orders*. London: Institute of Psychiatry.

Colombo, A., Bendelow, G., Fulford, K.W.M. and Williams, S. (2003) Model behaviour. *Openmind*, 125: 10–12.

Department for Constitutional Affairs (2007) *Mental Capacity Code of Practice 2005*. London: TSO.

Department of Health (1991) *The Patients' Charter*. London: Department of Health.

Department of Health (1999) *National Service Framework for Mental Health: Modern Standards and Service Models*. London: Department of Health.

Department of Health (2001) *Valuing People: A New Strategy for Learning Disability for the 21st Century*. London: Department of Health.

Department of Health (2007) *Service Users and Carers and the Care Programme Approach*. London: Department of Health.

Department of Health (2008) *Deprivation of Liberty Safeguards Code of Practice to Supplement the Main Mental Capacity Act 2005 Code of Practice*. London: TSO.

Department of Health (2009a) *Living Well with Dementia: A National Dementia Strategy*. London: Department of Health.

Department of Health (2009b) *Valuing People Now: A New Three Year Strategy for People with Learning Disabilities*. London: Department of Health.

Department of Health (2011) *No Health Without Mental Health*. London: Department of Health.

Department of Health/National Institute for Mental Health in England (2009) *The Legal Aspects of the Care and Treatment of Children and Young People with Mental Disorder: A Guide for Professionals*. London: Department of Health.

Dickenson, D. and Fulford, B. (2001) *In Two Minds: A Casebook of Psychiatric Ethics*. Oxford: Oxford University Press.

Emerson, E. et al. (2005) *The Impact of Person Centred Planning*. Lancaster: Institute of Health Research, Lancaster University.

Hale, B. (2010) *Mental Health Law*, 5th edn. London: Sweet and Maxwell.

HM Tribunals Service, *Mental Health Reports*.

Hope, T. (2004) *Medical Ethics: A Very Short Introduction*. Oxford: Oxford University Press.

Kitwood, T. (1997) *Dementia Reconsidered*. Milton Keynes: Open University Press.

Law Commission (1995) *Mental Incapacity*, Consultation Paper No. 231. London: HMSO.

Mental Health Foundation (2009) *Model Values?* London: Mental Health Foundation.

National Mental Health Development Unit (2009) *Independent Mental Health Advocacy: Effective Practice Guide*. London: Department of Health.

National Mental Health Development Unit (2009) *The Legal Aspects of the Care and Treatment of Children and Young People with Mental Disorder: A Guide for Professionals*. Available at: http://www.nmhdu.org.uk/silo/files/the-legal-aspects-of-the-care-and-treatment-of-children-and-young-people.pdf.

NHS Information Centre (2011) *Inpatients Formally Detained in Hospitals Under the Mental Health Act 1983 and Patient Subject to Supervised Community Treatment*, England 2011–12.

North East London NHS Trust (2010) *Mental Health Services Named Nurse Policy*.

Nursing and Midwifery Council (2008) *Code of Professional Conduct*. London: NMC.

Office for National Statistics (2005)

Priebe, S., Katsakou, C., Amos, T., Leese, M., Morriss, R., Rose, D., Wykes, T., Yeeles, K. (2009) Patients' views and read missions 1 year after involuntary hospitalisation. *British Journal of Psychiatry*, 194:1.

RCN (2009) *Mental Health in Children and Young People: An RCN Toolkit for Nurses Who Are Not Mental Health Specialists*. London: RCN.

Read, J. (2009) *Psychiatric Drugs: Key Issues and Service User Perspectives*. Basingstoke: Palgrave Macmillan.

Royal College of Psychiatrists (2008) *Fair Deal Manifesto*. London: RCP.

Royal College of Psychiatrists (2009) *Rethinking Risk to Others*, CR 151. London: RCP.

Shepherd, G., Boardman, G. and Slade, M. (2008) *Making Recovery a Reality*. London: Sainsbury Centre for Mental Health.

Slade, M. (2009) *100 Ways to Support Recovery: A Guide for Mental Health Professionals*. London: Rethink.

Social Exclusion Unit (2004) *Mental Health and Social Exclusion*. London: Social Exclusion Unit, Office of the Deputy Prime Minister.

Wilkinson, R. and Caulfield, H. (2000) *The Human Rights Act: A Practical Guide for Nurses*. London: Whurr.

Woodbridge, K. and Fulford, B. (2004) *Whose Values?* London: Sainsbury Centre for Mental Health.

Zigmond, A. (2010) *A Clinician's Brief Guide to the Mental Health Act*, 2nd ed. London: RCPsych Publications.

Index

Locators shown in *italics* refer to boxes, scenarios and tables.